SUPERVI

IN AUDIOLOGY

Supervision in Audiology by **Judith A. Rassi, M.A.** is a volume in the new **PERSPECTIVES IN AUDIOLOGY SERIES**—Lyle L. Lloyd, Ph.D., series editor. Other volumes in this series are:

Published:

Communicating with Deaf People: A Resource Manual for Teachers and Students of American Sign Language by Harry W. Hoemann, Ph.D.

Language Development and Intervention with the Hearing Impaired by Richard R. Kretschmer, Ed.D., and Laura W. Kretschmer, Ed.D.

Noise and Audiology edited by David M. Lipscomb, Ph.D.

Auditory Management of Hearing-Impaired Children: Principles and Prerequisites for Intervention edited by Mark Ross, Ph.D. and Thomas G. Giolas, Ph.D.

In preparation:

Elements of Hearing Science edited by Lawrence J. Deutsch, Ph.D., and Alan M. Richards, Ph.D.

Psychology of Deafness by Harry W. Hoemann, Ph.D.

Rehabilitative Audiology (Part I: The Adult/Part II: The Elderly Client) edited by Raymond H. Hull, Ph.D.

Introduction to Instrumental Phonetics by Colin Painter, Ph.D.

A Primer of Acoustic Phonetics by J. M. Pickett, Ph.D.

Hearing Assessment edited by William F. Rintelmann, Ph.D.

American Sign Language and Sign Systems by Ronnie Bring Wilbur, Ph.D.

Publisher's Note
Perspectives in Audiology is a carefully planned series of clinically oriented, topic-specific textbooks. The series is enriched by contributions from leading specialists in audiology and allied disciplines. Because technical language and terminology in these disciplines are constantly being refined and sometimes vary, this series has been edited as far as possible for consistency of style in conformity with current majority usage as set forth by the American Speech and Hearing Association, the *Publication Manual of the American Psychological Association,* and *The University of Chicago Manual of Style.* University Park Press and the series editors and authors welcome readers' comments about individual volumes in the series or the series concept as a whole in the interest of making **Perspectives in Audiology** as useful as possible to students, teachers, clinicians, and scientists.

A Volume in the Perspectives in Audiology Series

SUPERVISION IN AUDIOLOGY

Judith A. Rassi, M.A.

Associate in Audiology and Associate Director,
Northwestern University Medical School Hearing Clinic

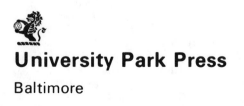

University Park Press

Baltimore

UNIVERSITY PARK PRESS
International Publishers in Science and Medicine
233 East Redwood Street
Baltimore, Maryland 21202

Copyright © 1978 by University Park Press

Typeset by American Graphic Arts Corporation.
Manufactured in the United States of America by The Maple Press Company.

Library of Congress Cataloging in Publication Data
Rassi, Judith A., 1939–
Supervision in audiology.

(Perspectives in audiology series)
Bibliography: p.
Includes indexes.
1. Audiology—Study and teaching—Supervision.
I. Title. II. Series. [DNLM: 1. Teaching.
2. Audiology—Education. WV18 R2228s]
RF291.R37   617.8'9'07   78-5701
ISBN 0-8391-1276-9

CONTENTS

PREFACE TO PERSPECTIVES IN AUDIOLOGY

Audiology is a young, vibrant, dynamic field. Its lineage can be traced to the fields of education, medicine, physics, and psychology in the nineteenth century and the emergence of speech pathology in the first half of this century. The term "audiology," meaning the science of hearing, was coined by Raymond Carhart in 1947. Since then, its definition has expanded to include its professional nature. Audiology is the profession that provides knowledge and service in the areas of human hearing and, more broadly, human communication and its disorders. As evidence of the growth of audiology as a major profession, in the 1940s there were no programs designed to prepare "audiologists," while now there are over 112 graduate training programs accredited by the Education and Training Board of the American Board of Examiners in Speech Pathology and Audiology for providing academic and clinical training designed to prepare clinically competent audiologists. Audiology is also a major area of study in the professional preparation of speech pathologists, speech and hearing scientists, and otologists.

Perspectives in Audiology is the first series of books designed to cover the major areas of study in audiology. The interdisciplinary nature of the field is reflected by the scope of the volumes in this series. The volumes currently in preparation (see p. ii) include both clinically oriented and basic science texts. The series consists of topic-specific textbooks designed to meet the needs of today's advanced level student. Each volume will also serve as a focal reference source for practicing audiologists and specialists in many related fields.

The **Perspectives in Audiology** series offers several advantages not usually found in other texts, but purposely featured in this series to increase the practical value of the books for practitioners and researchers, as well as for students and teachers.

1. Every volume includes thorough discussion of all relevant clinical and/or research papers on each topic.
2. Every volume is organized in an educational format to serve as the main text or as one of the main texts for graduate and advanced undergraduate students in courses on audiology and/or other studies concerned with human communication and its disorders.
3. Unlike ordinary texts, **Perspectives in Audiology** volumes will retain their professional reference value as focal reference sources for practitioners and researchers in career work long after completion of their studies.
4. Each volume serves as a rich source of authoritative, up-to-date information and valuable reviews for specialists in many fields, including administration, audiology, early childhood studies, linguistics, otology, psychology, pediatrics, public health, special education, speech pathology, and speech and hearing science.

Most audiologists today are, as most have been in the past, involved in the delivery of service. As professional preparation programs have developed in audiology, a heavy emphasis on practicum experience has concurrently developed. This emphasis has not thus far been met with a comprehensive, specialized text. *Supervision in Audiology,* by Judith A. Rassi, is the first and only book dealing exclusively with this topic and is therefore presented as an early volume in the **Perspectives in Audiology** series. Although other texts and significant portions of texts in speech pathology are concerned with supervision, this volume deals directly with the unique problems of supervision in the area of audiologic assessment. Clear and well organized methods of supervision geared to the specialized techniques and approaches of clinical training programs in audiology, are greatly needed, and Rassi has developed this text to answer that need.

Although the volume is designed primarily for the audiologic assessment clinical practicum, many of the concepts, particularly those in Chapter 4, and procedures described are directly applicable to supervision in other clinical areas. Habilitative and educational aspects of audiology are not emphasized because the available literature on supervision in speech pathology and in student teaching can provide the appropriate resource material. *Supervision in Audiology* is both a text for advanced students in audiology developing supervisory skills and a resource volume for supervisors of audiology practica. It is designed to enhance the quality of audiology practica experiences and thereby ultimately result in improved services to hearing impaired persons.

Lyle L. Lloyd, Ph.D.
Chairman and Professor of
Special Education
Professor of Audiology and
Speech Sciences
Purdue University

PREFACE

As a specific topic of discussion and investigation, supervision in audiology has been overlooked throughout its years of existence. Audiology supvervisors seeking to improve the quality of their work must depend largely on self-reliance. Such a nonsystem for professional training and growth is clearly undesirable. The informational vacuum in audiology supervision thus gave me reason to undertake this writing. Primarily, the material herein is based on my experience as a supervisor in audiology: on analyses of the supervisory process from within, on comments made by other supervisors, and on the many observations and reactions of students. These sources of input admittedly have generated more questions, frustrations, and concerns than answers or solutions; however, they have succeeded in motivating me to crystallize some of my thoughts on the supervisory tasks I confront daily. I am hopeful that the resultant statements in this book will lead the way for other supervisors in audiology to engage in self-evaluation and to examine their positions on issues of common concern. Once this hoped-for response has occurred, perhaps we will witness some discussion of this important topic in professional meetings as well as in the literature.

On many fronts, knowledge in the field of audiology is expanding so rapidly that the challenge to keep abreast of new developments can be overwhelming to any clinician. For a clinical supervisor, the implications of change are even more consequential, because he is directly responsible for demonstrating/teaching the latest advances in clinical knowhow to students. This added demand is compounded by yet another factor, the unending need for refinement of his supervisory techniques. It follows that continuing education for the supervisor in audiology must encompass both subject matter (the stuff of audiology) and teaching methods (clinical supervision). Both are available, though in somewhat disproportionate amounts. Unfortunately, these elements have not been offered in combination. Efforts need to focus on supervision as it is uniquely applied in the training of clinical audiologists. Specificity is essential if our successive aims are to improve audiology supervision, to prepare students for an unsettled, demanding field, and to promote good audiology.

In Chapter 1 of this book, the communicative disorders view of clinical supervision is discussed in historical terms, and then related to current needs in audiology. The many facets of audiology supervision and the audiology supervisor are considered in Chapters 2 and 3, respectively. Chapter 4 comprises a manual of methodology, and Chapter 5 describes a training program in audiology supervision.[1] A critical look at some of the issues facing university supervisors in speech pathology and audiology training programs is presented in Chapter 6.

Judith A. Rassi

---

[1] Supervision of aural rehabilitation aspects of audiology is not addressed in this text because it so closely parallels supervision of the kind of therapy involved in speech pathology work. Interested readers will find the many speech pathology supervision references cited herein more relevant and applicable.

ACKNOWLEDGMENTS

The writing of this text would not have been possible without inspiration from those who directly or indirectly shared the supervisory experience with me. To all such persons—patients, students, fellow supervisors, classroom instructors, administrators—I am grateful. And to those individuals who have actively participated in the Northwestern University audiology supervision training program, I offer express thanks; it is in this unique climate where the most deliberative considerations have been nurtured. The participants, too numerous to list here, have proven conclusively that audiology supervision is substantial, involved, and open to study. The persons who contributed materially are acknowledged in Appendix VI, the document they helped to prepare.

Three people devoted their personal time and energy to this effort. Jeanne Thomas Hugg provided ancillary support in the initial supervision training course offered to students. Special appreciation is also due Indiana University's Jean L. Anderson, a pioneer in communicative disorders supervision, who graciously agreed to review this material from her particular vantage point. Douglas Noffsinger's contribution has been singular. As my overseer, he authorized the reduction of my ordinary workload to allow writing time. Moreover, he gave unqualified support to the development of our supervision training program in all its facets. As my primary critic, Douglas Noffsinger showed unparalleled judgment in his tireless editing of the words on these pages. As my mentor, his advice throughout this venture has been astute and practical. And as my friend, his encouragement has been consistently reassuring.

SUPERVISION IN AUDIOLOGY

CHAPTER 1

INTRODUCTION

CONTENTS

The field of speech pathology and audiology is widely recognized as a clinical discipline. Although the academic and research components of our field play equally important roles in the study of communicative disorders, each is directly related to the substance of clinical endeavors. The preponderance of coursework in our training programs is devoted to the analysis of speech, hearing, and language problems, their ramifications, and the clinical approaches designed for their remediation. Likewise, the major thrust of many research efforts is the investigation of clinical manifestations endemic to the communicatively impaired and, ultimately, the refinement of clinical techniques. It thus becomes imperative for both the classroom instructor and the clinical researcher, as well as the clinician, to acquire a working knowledge of clinical procedures.

University training programs traditionally have attempted to uphold this worthy goal through curricular and clinical practicum offerings. The American Speech and Hearing Association (ASHA) requirements for the Certificates of Clinical Competence (CCC; Asha, 1975c) served to reinforce such efforts to upgrade the quality of our profession. Indeed, the CCC requirements, including the important Clinical Fellowship Year, have been fulfilled by many individuals who aspired to be instructors, administrators, and/or researchers rather than clinicians. Although the incentive to obtain the CCC for these persons may be employment (the CCC is now a common prerequisite for employment in our field, regardless of the specific job description), the desired end result has been achieved through certification requirements. That is to say, all CCC holders must have gained a certain amount of clinical expertise before launching their respective careers. In addition, the recent definitive statement of minimum requirements for accreditation of education and training programs issued by the ASHA Educational and Training Board (Asha, 1976a, 1976b) reflects even greater effort in the area of quality control. Programs seeking accreditation are directed to comply with precepts in a number of areas, each of which is a vital ingredient in the maintenance of optimum professional training.

Although the adoption of such standards by ASHA has helped promote the goal of providing well trained, well prepared speech and language pathologists and audiologists, the attainment of this goal remains a hit-and-miss venture. And the reason is clear: the core of the professional training program, clinical practicum, has not been sufficiently explored. Despite stipulations regarding numbers of clinical clock hours, diversity in settings and clientele, clinical certification of supervisors, and amount of direct supervision, there have been no specific guidelines for the supervisor to heed (Anderson, 1975). Furthermore, no one has systematically analyzed the supervisory process in our field (Engnoth and Lingwall, 1974). We have yet to identify precisely those intangible attributes that separate "good" supervisors from "bad" supervisors. And because we have not determined what it is that constitutes excellence in a supervised clinical experience, we have largely ignored the training of supervisors. In short, we are not certain *who* should be supervising our students-in-training, *what* such persons should be doing to effect learning in the clinical setting, *when* they need assistance in their work, *where* there are needs for improvement of technique, and *why* present supervisors are doing whatever it is that they do. With increasing demands for accountability in all facets of our profession, intensive examination of these basic questions is long overdue (Anderson, 1973b).

The lack of research in this area is ironic given the fact that our profession's collective effectiveness is dependent on the success of clinical training procedures. A tenable supposition is that training programs are only as strong as the clinical practicum element within them and that clinical practicum, in turn, is only as effective as the competencies of participating supervisors. It therefore behooves us to unravel the mysteries of supervision.

BACKGROUND

Recognition of the need for investigation of supervision in communicative disorders is not new. In 1963, participants of the ASHA-sponsored National Conference on Graduate Education in Speech Pathology and Audiology supported resolutions calling for higher recognition of faculty-supervisors and improvement of their status to levels accorded academic and research persons (Darley, 1963). The following year, a seminar on Guidelines for Supervision of Clinical Practicum in Programs of Training for Speech Pathologists and Audiologists was conducted by ASHA (Villareal, 1964). This study group examined supervision with unprecedented thoroughness, citing issues of concern and calling "attention to the need for objective evidence to support experienced judgment" (Villareal, p. 35) in supervisory matters such as the evaluation of students and the selection and training of supervisors. At another 1964 conference sponsored by ASHA, Guidelines for the Internship Year, participants stressed the importance of exploring the clinical supervision area and recommended that supervision training be initiated in speech pathology and audiology (Kleffner, 1964).

As evidenced by articles published in the 1960s, this period also marked the beginning of individual concern over the quality of clinical supervision. [Earlier writings dealt exclusively with supervision of student teaching in the public schools (Anderson, 1973b).] In general, the second-generation authors addressed the need for upgrading supervision (Darley, 1969; Miner, 1967; Ward and Webster, 1965b) and the training of supervisors (Halfond, 1964; Stace and Drexler, 1969), student/supervisor interactions (Ingram and Stunden, 1967; Miner, 1967; Van Riper, 1965; Ward and Webster, 1965a, 1965b), evaluation of student clinicians' performance (Miner, 1967; Rees and Smith, 1967, 1968), and desirable/undesirable supervisory approaches (Erickson and Van Riper, 1967; Van Riper and Dopheide, 1966; Ward and Webster, 1965a, 1965b). Although some of this material continued to focus on supervision in the schools, university clinical training programs per se received more attention.

With the 1970s came more articles and conference reports of increasingly substantive nature. Two group undertakings, a conference on Supervision of Speech and Hearing Programs in the Public Schools (Anderson, 1970) and a workshop on Supervision in Speech Pathology (Turton, 1973), yielded extensive published accounts of their proceedings. Surveys were conducted to explore the status of supervision and practicum in the schools by the ASHA Task Force on Supervision in the Schools (Brown et al., 1972) and by the Council of College and University Supervisors of Practicum in the Schools, an organization founded in 1970 (Anderson, 1973a). Individuals also polled supervisors (Anderson, 1972; Schubert and Aitchison, 1975) as well as graduates (Culatta, Colucci, and Wiggins, 1975) regarding their views on training needs and the supervisory process. Several authors presented information on specific methodologies in supervision, such as evaluation procedures (Klevans and Volz, 1974; Shriberg et al., 1975b), use of behavior modification as a training technique (Starkweather, 1974), and conference analysis (Boone and Prescott, 1972; Culatta and Seltzer, 1976; Culatta and Seltzer, 1977). A handbook on supervision in speech pathology also became available (Oratio, 1977).

Accompanying the growing number of publications and conferences have been convention papers, seminars, and workshops on supervision. Indeed, a supervisor may now attend a convention session devoted entirely to papers dealing with supervision. Furthermore, such presentations are being offered at professional meetings on national, regional, state, and local levels. Quite naturally, this burgeoning interest has resulted in the development of university courses on supervision.

As a consequence of our field's maturation in this area, the Council of College and University Supervisors of Practicum in the Schools changed its name in 1974 to the Council of University Supervisors of Practicum in Speech Pathology and Audiology, thereby expanding its membership to include all clinical supervisors (Asha, 1975a). Concurrently, the ASHA Legislative Council established a Committee on Supervision in Speech Pathology and Audiology (Asha, 1975b), charging it to "study the status of supervision of speech pathology and audiology as it relates to the entire profession in training programs, the Clinical Fellowship Year, and employment settings" (Asha, 1975d, p. 397). These actions took place at the 1974 ASHA Convention. This productive year also saw the appearance of an article by Schubert (1974) in which minimal requirements for clinical supervisors were suggested.

Past and present efforts represent only a modest beginning, however. As noted in several writings (Anderson, 1970, 1973b; Brown, 1967; Halfond, 1964) and convention presentations (Anderson, 1975; Brown, 1975), supervision has been thoroughly and systematically investigated in other areas, such as business management, psychology, social work, and teacher education. Although the resultant publications in these fields do not have direct application to supervision in communicative disorders, they have much to offer on topics pertinent to any type of supervision, for example, interpersonal relationships, competency-based instruction, and leadership techniques. A sampling of materials presented by professionals outside our field, then, can be quite rewarding for the supervisor seeking expert guidance, especially if that person is skillful in adapting ideas to suit his own needs. A wealth of information is also available to those speech and language pathologists and audiologists whose research interests encompass supervision, for example, as in Blumberg (1974), Cogan (1973), Goldhammer (1969), and Unruh and Turner (1970). Notwithstanding their usefulness, such outside resource materials make it clear that the communicative disorders sector has barely begun its search. Perhaps our field's growing interest in supervision will now bring us to a stage of similarly serious analysis and research commitment.

SPEECH AND LANGUAGE PATHOLOGY VS. AUDIOLOGY

Conspicuous by its absence in virtually every presentation on supervision in our field is any mention of supervision in audiology per se. Although many references are made to "speech and language pathology and audiology," "speech pathology and audiology," or "speech and hearing," the accompanying text does not really address itself to audiology. It would be a mistake to assume that supervision of clinical practicum in speech and language pathology is so similar to that in audiology that the two can be treated in the same way. Even though these branches of our field have common supervision components, there are more differences than there are similarities between the actual supervisory processes.

Although a search of the literature reveals one article which touches on supervision in audiology, the essence of that report is a general description of aural rehabilitation practicum in a training program (Erickson and Garstecki, 1973). In other words, there is no focus on specific supervisory techniques or on the vast array of audiologic procedures which are not therapy oriented. For the supervisor of audiology practicum, then, there is nothing available that is directly applicable to his specialty. His only recourse is to adapt information on supervision from the speech and language pathology areas along with that which comes from other professional disciplines.

A simple comparison of commonly used clinical procedures in speech and language pathology to those employed by audiologists will serve to illustrate some basic differences in clinical approach, differences that necessitate dissimilar approaches to supervision. The magnitude of disparity between these factions, of course, depends on the modus operandi of the clinical programs being compared. Nonetheless, some generalizations are in order for the purpose of isolating those major differences that have implications in the supervisory process. For example:

SPEECH AND LANGUAGE PATHOLOGY	AUDIOLOGY
A. *Premise*	A. *Premise*
Ongoing therapy sessions follow diagnostic workup. Student is likely to see a given patient repeatedly.	Evaluation, recommendation, and referral are often accomplished in one or two clinic sessions. Student is likely to see a given patient only one time. Due to the nature of practicum assignments, this likelihood exists even when patients return for followup visits (unless aural rehabilitation practicum is assigned).
Implications for supervision	*Implications for supervision*
1. Pre-therapy lesson plans can be outlined by student and/or supervisor.	1. Pre-test session information is often limited, if not unavailable, for planning purposes.

2. Supervisor can review errors, make suggestions to student for change after each session, if desired, to be implemented by the student during ensuing sessions. Thus, student mistakes are often not *immediately* critical.

2. Supervisor must make suggestions, corrections during the course of an audiologic evaluation. Thus, student mistakes are often *immediately* critical.

3. Rapport between student and patient can be developed over time.

3. Rapport between student and patient must be successfully established within one session.

4. Recommendations and referrals can be formulated over time, if desired, on the basis of therapy results, thereby allowing such decision making to be protracted.

4. Recommendations and referrals are usually immediate, thus forcing quick, consequential decision making.

5. Student may work with no more than several patients during a school-term clinical assignment, thus limiting the variety of case types he will see within this time period. Supervision is focused accordingly.

5. Student works with many different patients in a clinical assignment, thus making it possible for him to see a wide variety of case types within a given assignment. Supervision must be broad in scope.

B. *Premise*

Although test equipment may be frequently utilized, it is relatively uncomplicated and limited in variety.

B. *Premise*

A wide array of sophisticated test equipment, including hearing aids, is basic to audiologic evaluation. Test procedures are often technically complex.

Implication for supervision

The student's acquisition of technical knowhow is of secondary importance in clinical practicum.

Implication for supervision

The operation of test equipment and modification of test procedures via equipment manipulation constitute a major part of clinical work.

These comparisons should not be misconstrued as an attempt to diminish the complexity of speech and language pathology practica while inflating the importance of clinical audiology. One could easily compile another comparative set of clinical activities that would highlight more involved components of speech and language pathology clinical work, and then contrast them to relatively uncomplicated audiology tasks. Rather, as already stated, the parallels drawn here have been selected to emphasize the necessity of differing modes of supervision.

Although basic differences in approach may seem obvious to many supervisors, close inspection of audiology training programs would likely uncover arbitrary combinations of actual supervisory procedures. Today's supervisors in audiology, because of the lack of training specifically designed to prepare them for their unique teaching roles, are using tools inherited from their predecessors. As Anderson (1975) so aptly said: "We supervise as we were supervised. Information is handed down as folklore." This unfortunate situation applies to all supervisors without training, but it probably has the most negative impact on the audiology supervisors. A look at the history of our field is enlightening in this regard.

Two factors in the development of speech pathology and audiology as clinical entities have contributed to the status of supervision in audiology: (1) speech pathology as a field preceded audiology by many years; and (2) audiology, the offspring of many disciplines, has a dominant genesis in speech pathology. Furthermore, many audiologists did their undergraduate work in speech pathology before they pursued graduate training in audiology. As a result, those persons who pioneered supervision in audiology were necessarily influenced by speech pathology approaches in clinical practice and supervision technique. Given the absence of specific training in audiology supervision, it is reasonable to conclude that this set of circumstances is still effective today. That is to say, supervision in audiology, having no strong image of its own, continues to be patterned unduly after supervision in speech pathology.

The perpetuation of unmethodical supervision planning in audiology can be viewed from another perspective. Many audiologists who are now functioning as supervisors had poorly-prepared supervisor models: doctoral students with little or no on-the-job clinical experience (Rosen, 1967); classroom instructors whose primary function was an academic rather than clinical role; and/or persons who had much more clinical experience in speech pathology than they did in audiology, even though they may have had ASHA certification in both areas. It is not uncommon for audiology graduates to report that their clinical practicum was not closely supervised and that they were allowed to see patients with no more than cursory monitoring by the supervisor assigned to them. Although ETB regulations (Asha, 1976a, 1976b) are doing much to rectify this situation, the fact remains that many audiology students are still being prepared for their careers by supervisors who are largely unprepared for theirs.

These statements are not being postulated to indict all supervision in audiology. Undoubtedly, there are many dedicated supervisors who work diligently to upgrade the quality of their supervision, and a significant number probably succeed in their efforts. However, such achievements are essentially unguided and solely dependent on personal ingenuity. In view of this situation, we need to capitalize on the groundwork laid by our colleagues in speech pathology and in other fields. We must adapt it to our own needs, however, and thereupon build a body of knowledge and technique that is uniquely applicable to supervision in audiology. It is not enough to model our clinical teaching after a field that is similar to our own, yet has distinct differences. It is not enough to expect our supervisors to be skilled in their roles when their preparation has been nonexistent, inappropriate, or haphazard. And it is not enough to hope that our students' supervised clinical practicum experiences will somehow "work out for the best" when there are available means to analyze, structure, and control this critically important aspect of our training programs. The field of audiology has matured to the point at which it can no longer afford to leave its vital core training to chance.

CHAPTER 2

THE COMPOSITION OF SUPERVISION IN AUDIOLOGY

CONTENTS

There are probably as many definitions of supervision as there are supervisors. As Anderson (1975) points out, one's own definition is based on, and affected by, how one supervises. The literature supports her observation. That being so, I herewith offer my own definition of supervision, one which generally describes my function as a clinical supervisor of audiology students in a graduate training program:

> Clinical supervision is clinical teaching. Its aim is to teach a student in a one-to-one situation how to apply his academic knowledge in a practical clinical setting as he functions in that setting. The ultimate goal is to transform the student into an independent clinician.

Anderson (1973b; 1975) views supervision as a role having many components, only one of which is teaching. Some of the other important aspects of supervision, as she identifies them, are: leadership, communication, interpersonal relationships, analysis, facilitation, management, and evaluation. Supervision in audiology embraces all of these components, although I prefer to schematize it in such a way that clinical teaching is singled out as *the* role, with the others being integral, contributing factors.

Clinical supervision is a complex process. It involves a type of teaching that differs markedly from the lecture/listen and group discussion formats of formally taught courses and seminars. And although it may bear some resemblance to a one-to-one tutorial exchange between teacher and student, it represents a significant departure from this practice also. A fundamental difference, of course, is the participation of a third person, the patient, or possibly more persons if the patient's family is included. Each of the participants in this triad—supervisor, student clinician, and patient—must understand his role, and the dynamics of the resultant interaction are extremely complicated and variable, as noted by Halfond (1964, p. 442). Another variation on the

9

traditional classroom paradigm is the learning-by-doing nature of clinical practicum, a characteristic that likens it to the laboratory instruction models common to many fields in the arts and sciences as well as to the professions. To Anderson, this makes it "a very special kind of teaching—perhaps the best kind," in that the clinical teacher "has the advantage of a very special situation in which the student can really learn by doing" (1973b, p. 17).

It is the learning-by-doing feature that poses a unique challenge to the audiology supervisor, because clinical supervision in audiology must necessarily transcend the teaching of theory application. Regardless of the quality of accompanying classroom instruction in clinically oriented audiology courses, it is virtually impossible to prepare a student for the infinite variety of clinical testing problems he will face in his clinical practicum assignments. Obviously, the broad range of patients' behavioral idiosyncrasies cannot be anticipated in didactic instruction. Likewise, without actual hearing-impaired subjects in the classroom, one cannot teach in advance the gamut of possible variations in clinically demonstrated auditory behavior, such as intertest discrepancies, masking enigmas, and irreconcilable hearing aid performance scores. The "textbook cases" are thus limited in scope and number. Indeed, a student may encounter in his clinical practicum experience a substantial number of cases that are incongruent with the more straightforward, classical examples he has learned about in class. And no amount of practice on a programmed simulator and/or on normal hearing subjects can adequately prepare a beginning student for the real world of hearing-impaired human beings.

Next, there are some audiologic concepts that at least a few students never seem to learn well in the classroom. Interestingly, a student sometimes performs well academically, as revealed by examinations and grades, yet may not fully understand what he seemingly mastered in his coursework. Or, there is the student who simply produces work of overall mediocre quality. Both types may need the practical, individualized teaching provided by clinical instruction to enhance learning. Finally, the integration of knowledge often does not occur in a student's mind until he has had the opportunity to see informational factors converge and interact in the practical embodiment of patient, test findings, and clinical environment.

And so there is a clear need to expand any definition/description of supervision in audiology, taking into account not only application of theory, but also the extension and refinement of learning, as well as the practical integration of classroom-imparted information. Such teaching can only take place in a clinical setting. Moreover, clinical teaching not only supplements classroom teaching, it complements classroom teaching. One mode of instruction would not be meaningful without the other. Although it is tempting to refer to the content of classroom teaching as the "what" of audiology and the substance of clinical teaching as the "how" of audiology, there is too much overlap between the two to render them mutually exclusive. Nonetheless, it is in the clinic where the student clinician serves his apprenticeship and actually learns to use the tools of his trade. It is in the clinic where he learns to cope with the multitude of variables which exist in everday audiologic endeavors. And only the clinical teacher, or supervisor, is in a position to make the adage, "experience is the best teacher," become a truism for each student; only the supervisor can help the student learn by doing.

COMPETENCY-BASED INSTRUCTION

Supervision has been defined in two ways thus far: by identifying its components, as enumerated by Anderson, and by distinguishing its practical teaching characteristics. The latter analysis leads naturally to another way in which clinical supervision can be viewed; that is, as a skill-building task or as competency-based instruction. Anderson has described competency-based instruction as "the establishment of precise objectives and accountability for meeting those objectives" (1974, p. 9). To dissect audiology supervision in this manner, one must first isolate those clinical activities that, when grouped together, may be identified as worthwhile competencies to be pursued. From this, a precise quantification of audiology supervision should begin to emerge.

The schematic depiction in Figure 1 represents one way in which the skills or competencies of a clinical audiologist might be delineated. It should be noted that this diagram has been labeled "skill/competency scales" in accordance with the attempt to rank items in order of difficulty. This has been accomplished by arranging the columns—testing, writing, interpersonal, and decision making—from left to right in a sequence of assumed progressive difficulty. In like manner, the clinical skills within each category are stacked in columnar formation to denote increasingly higher levels of performance. Each column is also flanked by the phrases "with supervision" on the left and "without supervision" on the right, to indicate that the listed competencies, when placed in a supervision context, must first be taught to the student before he can be expected to demonstrate a proficiency that warrants departure of the supervisor. The desired end product of such a supervision process appears at the top of this chart: the student who is sufficiently competent to assume the responsibilities of independent patient management.

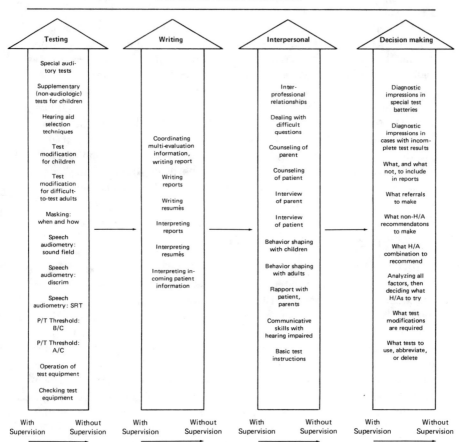

Figure 1.   Skill/Competency Scales

As any audiologist will recognize, these skill/competency scales are by no means all-inclusive. They are not intended to be so. Such a goal is probably unachievable because the duties of audiologists can vary among clinicians, work settings, and training programs, depending largely on the philosophical orientation of each. Also, one could easily examine audiologic competencies in much greater detail than is shown here. Again, variations in clinical approach would dictate the substance and method of such an analysis. Moreover, an exacting breakdown seems unnecessary for the purpose of this discussion. The scales, then, merely illustrate a general view of audiology supervision within the framework of competency-based instruction.

An experienced supervisor might understandably debate the sequential order of difficulty gradation in the scales. This is to be expected, because there is often no distinct demarcation between degrees of difficulty in these tasks. Their potential overlap is a direct consequence of the peculiarities of the patient and the strengths and weaknesses of the student. For example: a student may be very adept at report writing but unable to operate equipment smoothly; or, perhaps, a student may work more easily with children than with adults; or, in one case, the patient may be difficult to counsel and easy to test, while in another, just the reverse may be true.

The order of difficulty assigned to these competencies further suggests a possible sequence for their presentation in clinical instruction. Even if this sequence were considered to be ideal, however, its enactment would be impractical if not impossible. Unfortunately, one cannot schedule certain portions of an audiologic evaluation just for the students' sake. Such fragmentation of patient service is obviously inadvisable. The supervisor should not seriously compromise the evaluation of patients to match the skills of a student at a given moment. This situation inevitably imposes certain constraints on both the student clinician and his clinical supervisor, constraints which, incidentally, are not faced in classroom instruction.

For the supervisor, the intercurrence of complex cases in the practicum sequence of a beginning student clinician leaves but one course of action: the student must necessarily be exposed to competencies he is not yet expected to master. Little time and effort need be wasted, however, as the supervisor should see in each case a rich source of teaching points. Even though he may not permit the student to participate fully in the workup of a case, the supervisor can and should seize the opportunity to make each clinical experience as meaningful as possible for the student. This can be accomplished by the supervisor's serving as a model for the student while simultaneously providing continuous (insofar as possible) explanatory narration. Following the audiologic evaluation, the supervisor can amplify on salient points. If time restrictions interfere with this procedure, even the briefest of explanations will serve the student in some way. Although circumstances may be forcing the student to revert temporarily to the role of observer, much learning can still take place.

The important point to make here is that the student may never again have another opportunity during his graduate training program to see a case like the current one. Hence, the supervisor cannot afford to gloss over valuable teaching material. At the same time, the student needs to be accumulating a store of cases in his mind for future recall. It is to be hoped that, at a later, more advanced stage in his training, he will be able to look back on some of his previous clinical experiences and learn from them again. In the matter of specific test skills to which the student might be exposed prematurely, assimilation of the rudiments can at least begin. As will be discussed later, repeated exposure to all clinical activities provides the reinforcement so necessary for learning. And the sooner the exposure begins, the more samples the student is likely to see.

If the overlapping of competencies is sometimes trying for the supervisor, it can be equally so for the student. For some, it is quite confusing, even if the supervisor has done his utmost to structure the teaching situation as much as possible. For others, it seems to make little difference, as they are capable of acquiring competencies and synthesizing information regardless of the order of presentation. Clearly, there are some students who naturally learn faster than others. A big factor in the sequencing of competencies is the sequencing of clinical assignments, an issue that is considered in Chapter 4.

LEVELS OF SUPERVISION

Supervision in audiology can be examined from yet another angle. Having defined the process, one needs to look at the various supervisory approaches that are available to the audiology supervisor. These can be termed appropriately at levels of supervision because they entail a hierarchy. And their design, as specified both by composition and ordered arrangement, allows for a rather direct application to the previously described skill/competency scales.

Before selecting the level(s) of supervision to be employed, the supervisor should have some foreknowledge of the student's background and skills. As this determination is made, the following factors need to be considered: the student's academic preparation; whether or not he has had previous clinical assignments and, if so, the type, number, and duration of these assignments, and the quality of his work (that is, his strengths and weaknesses) in said assignments. Such preliminary information will give the supervisor at least a general impression of an incoming student's capabilities, thereby forming the basis for a tentative decision on the initial supervisory approach. The supervisor will not be able to make a firm judgment, however, until he actually has had the opportunity to observe and work with the student several times. Then, when a clearer picture of the student's clinical skills emerges along with his working relationship with the supervisor, the latter will have a more informed opinion and can choose the level(s) of supervision accordingly.

A roster of feasible levels of supervision in audiology is herewith presented, starting first with the approach to be used with the most inexperienced clinician, then gradually progressing to levels suitable for more advanced students:

1. Detailed explanation, with accompanying demonstration, of every action from beginning to end of test session
2. General explanation, with some accompanying demonstration, of every action from beginning to end of test session
3. Suggestions or corrections while student is performing task(s) under close supervision
4. Prestructuring[1] of task(s) beforehand, with no explanation while student is performing task(s)
5. Instruction of student on what task is to be performed and its underlying rationale, but no explanation of how to do it before, during, or after task performance
6. Review beforehand with student of task(s) to be performed with student making all decisions; accompanying suggestions only when necessary
7. Review of task(s) with student only after he has completed them
8. Student makes all decisions, performs all tasks alone, with supervisory monitoring and suggestions only when deemed necessary

As can be seen, each succeeding level requires less active participation by the supervisor, while, at the same time, the student's direct involvement and attendant responsibilities increase. The objective in this sequence matches that previously displayed at the pinnacle of the skill/ competency scales; that is, student independence. Stated differently, the movement is from a supervisor-controlled situation to a student-controlled situation. Even so, it is important to note that the highest level does not permit exclusive control by the student because the supervisor is readily available for consultation.

At this point, it may be meaningful to examine the proposition of student independence in a supervised clinical situation. My own experience as a clinical supervisor in audiology has taught me that it is important to maintain some control of the proceedings regardless of how capable the student seems to be. This conclusion is based on two notions. First, it is essential that the supervisor know what is happening at all times, not because he lacks trust in the student's abilities, but because the patient is still the supervisor's responsibility. In most cases, it will be the supervisor, not the student, who controls followup patient management. Thus, it is the supervisor's duty as a responsible *clinician* to establish an identification bond with the patient and his presenting problems. Second,

---

[1] The term "prestructure" is used to describe the type of supervisory instruction that frequently precedes a clinical task and that includes a proposed, structured set of contingencies for the student to follow.

the supervisor, with his more extensive background of clinical experience, should be equipped to give even the most advanced student the benefit of his expertise on every case. In fact, it is the clinically mature student who often gains the most from any bonus clinical insights offered him. As a consequence, supervision at this level can be mutually stimulating, hence most rewarding for both parties.

Although student independence is a desirable goal, it appears to be in the best of interest of everyone concerned—supervisor, student, and patient—for the actual supervision process to be sustained. If this were not deemed necessary, one could grant students assignments without supervisors; and there is no indication of the desirability of such a revision in basic audiology training. Externships (discussed in Chapter 4) and the Clinical Fellowship Year have already been designed to provide appropriate settings for the more self-reliant type of supervised clinical work so important to the effective transition from student clinician to seasoned clinician.

Turning back to all the levels of supervision, one can see that the first seven are classifiable as teaching functions, while the label of supervision is warranted only for the eighth, and final, level. This designation of terms corresponds to the definition of supervision postulated at the beginning of this chapter. Whenever instruction is involved, teaching is occurring. It is only at the last stage, when the supervisor has reduced his participation to an advisory capacity, that the role becomes truly supervisory. Therefore, clinical supervision in audiology is largely a teaching task, or, at least, it should be. Some supervisors perform their duties primarily at the eighth level when they ought to be doing much more actual clinical teaching as typified by the other levels. Such inappropriate "remote-control" supervision must be changed, because it drastically shortchanges a student's clinical learning needs. And it certainly does not enhance the supervisor's image. Each supervisor must come to terms with the peculiar requirements of his/her job, and then adopt the most suitable type of supervisory approach(es) which satisfies those requirements (Mullendore and Koller, 1976).

SUPERVISION STATIONS

In connection with the aforementioned "remote-control" supervision (passive, noninvolved supervision from afar), it is important to consider the physical location of the audiology supervisor as he carries out his responsibilities to the student and patient. The following alternatives, listed in order from close proximity to the most distal placement, are

offered as reasonable teaching/supervisory stations.[2] They are conformable to the previously discussed levels of supervision:

1. Supervisor performing all tasks, simultaneously explaining his
    actions and underlying rationale as student observes; in other words,
    "supervisor in test chair."
2. Supervisor seated alongside student at all times, instructing him
    every step of the way.
3. Supervisor in test room with student during contact with patient (for
    example, placing earphones, conducting interview, doing counseling,
    choosing and trying on hearing aids).
4. Supervisor in control room to observe student's testing, giving sug-
    gestions and instruction when and where necessary.
5. Supervisor in control room, watching student through window and/
    or listening to him via talkback system, as student is in test room
    with patient.
6. Supervisor spot checks student's activities regularly and at strategic
    times throughout test session.
7. Supervisor monitors all testing and student-patient interaction from
    room adjacent to test/control rooms. Intervenes only when
    necessary.
8. Supervisor absent from premises. (Ideally, this should never occur.
    However, if circumstances compel such, the supervisor's absence
    should be limited to as brief a period as possible, and he should
    inform the student of his intention to leave as well as the time of his
    expected return. If the supervisor has a choice, the most logical time
    to make his exit is during an activity which he knows the student can
    handle somewhat independently.)

As implied in the eighth point, it is unacceptable for the supervisor
to desert the student and patient for extended periods of time. If student
errors are committed during such absences, valuable test time will have
been wasted unnecessarily. Examples of such time-consuming mistakes
are: "masking" during an entire pure tone testing sequence of one ear
with the masking unit inadvertently turned off; or testing complete
performance with a hearing aid turned to an inadequate volume setting.
As a consequence of such untimely-discovered errors, the patient will be
robbed of time and professional service when the supervisor is forced to

---

[2] Assignment of these stations was undertaken with the consideration of a clinical
facility having no special observation areas. Obviously, supervisor placement would be
somewhat altered, and certainly facilitated, by the presence of such areas.

sacrifice some other portion of the evaluation to accomplish the required retesting. Although a valid point may be made in favor of the "sink or swim" approach to supervision, in that a student will learn most retentively from his greatest errors, patient service should not be compromised. Again, the supervisor must remember his ever-present obligation to the patient, and then balance commitments accordingly.

COMPETENCY/LEVEL/STATION COMBINATIONS

An overall view of the levels of supervision and the related physical location points reveals some overlapping among the items in each list, similar to that observed in the skill/competency scales. This is to be expected, of course, if these three gauges of supervision correlate with one another. An intermixing of supervision levels with supervisor placements might be illustrated with two examples.

> A student may have proven that he is capable of performing basic audiometric testing rather independently (thus supervisor needs only spot check his testing, then review the final results), but he is nowhere near the stage of independence in hearing aid selection procedures (so supervisor must remain in test room with student during selection procedures).
> Another student may require minimal supervision throughout the actual test session (supervisor would conduct spot-checks and monitor student via talkback system), but the patient presents a complex counseling/management problem (supervisor may elect to do the patient counseling or, at the very least, provide considerable prestructuring for the student, and then monitor the student closely throughout the counseling session with intervention or followup if deemed appropriate).

It can thus be seen that the supervisor must continually assess the student's capabilities in order to determine what level(s) of supervision to use, and where to position himself during each activity. And the supervisor cannot assume that the student's progress, however consistent, will allow a smooth transition from level to level in an orderly sequence, because each case presents a new set of problems. Rather, it is important that he keep a close watch on the student's clinical strengths and weaknesses so that he will know at what points in an audiologic evaluation the student needs special help, and where the student can be allowed to work more independently. By the same token, the supervisor should note which types of clinical problems the student has encountered previously. This will enable him to ascertain whether or not the student is making progress in specific areas, hence whether or not supervisory approaches can be changed. The process demands ongoing watchfulness and accomodation.

CHAPTER 3

THE CLINICAL
SUPERVISOR IN AUDIOLOGY

CONTENTS

A discussion of the composition of supervision in audiology would be incomplete without giving searching consideration to the key element in the supervisory interaction, the supervisor. In a survey of clinical supervisors in college and university speech and hearing training programs, Schubert and Aitchison (1975) sought to profile the "typical" supervisor by analyzing such statistics as age, sex, salary, degree, position, preparation for supervision, and years of experience, as well as information about actual supervision. However, as subsequently pointed out by Shriberg et al. (1975a), the conclusions reached on the basis of these data were overgeneralized and distorted due to the inclusion of a large percentage of respondents whose primary responsibilities were something other than clinical supervision. Furthermore, no attempt was made to distinguish supervisors in speech pathology from those in audiology, though 7% of the respondents did report having a Certificate of Clinical Competence in Audiology, and 14% said they had dual certification.

There is little meaningful information on the audiology supervisor; therefore, it might be beneficial to look at what this person should be. That is to say, what characteristics does this person need in order to carry out effectively the responsibilities of such a multifaceted role? And how do these properties expressly qualify a person for the kinds of supervisory tasks involved in clinical audiology? As stated in the introductory chapter of this book, others have previously offered opinions on what individual attributes are desirable in a clinical supervisor, but no one has applied them to the unique requirements of audiology. Chapter 3 is therefore devoted to this end.

Because identification of suitable characteristics for the audiology supervisor is unprecedented, the groundwork initiated in speech pathology will help to serve this purpose. Accordingly, the following set of characteristics has been designed to take advantage of Anderson's components of supervision (1973b, 1975). Other fitting entries have been incorporated to make the outlined list more complete.

I.   Competencies
    A.   Master clinician
    B.   Teaching ability
       1.   Leadership
       2.   Communication
       3.   Interpersonal relationships
       4.   Analysis
       5.   Facilitation
       6.   Management
       7.   Evaluation

(Items B through 7 bracketed as: Anderson's eight components of supervision)

II. Qualities
    A.   Patience
    B.   Sense of humor
    C.   Commitment to clinical supervision
    D.   Interest in continued learning in audiology

As indicated, these characteristics can be divided somewhat logically into two categories: competencies—relatively extrinsic attainments that include definable, teachable elements (interpersonal relationships being a notable exception, though this, too, is largely dependent on external factors); and qualities—attributes of a more inherent, individually personal nature. In response to Anderson's charge that "the profession as a whole should begin to identify those competencies needed by all supervisors of the clinical process and those competencies needed in specific job environments . . ." (1974, p. 9), the listed competencies will be examined. Quite simply, there are two basic competency sets to be considered: clinical skills and teaching skills.

COMPETENCIES

Master Clinician

Excellent clinical skills, represented in this discussion by the familiar term, "master clinician," are clearly essential to high-quality supervision. Unless the supervisor knows his clinical job well and is capable of making, and carrying out, appropriate clinical decisions, he obviously is not prepared for a supervisory post. Without clinical expertise, how can he be expected to impart such wisdom to a student? An impressionable, clinically naive student should not receive misinformation from a supervisor, particularly during the indoctrination period of his practicum assignments. This is especially important because the student is not yet prepared to be a discerning judge of clinical ability. Not only can he acquire and internalize erroneous reasoning at this concept-developing stage, but poorly executed test techniques, if fostered and reinforced, may become deeply entrenched habits. If such misfortune befalls the student, he may or may not recover during subsequent, more enlightening supervised experiences. This is not to say that there is only one way to accomplish certain clinical goals, nor that all clinicians even seek the same goals. However, each clinician must draw from a body of knowledge comprised of accepted facts, and then function with workable clinical procedures. There are many options within this framework, but one must be sufficiently knowledgeable to make appropriate selections and implement them accordingly.

Despite its demands for clinical correctness, the "master clinician" stipulation cannot be interpreted to mean that a supervisor has all the answers. In an area like clinical audiology, answers are often not clearcut. The sensible supervisor, therefore, will tell the student when he is not certain the correct decision is being made, the reason for this uncertainty, and the rationale for selecting a strategy from a set of possible options. In fact, it is part of the supervisor's teaching obligation to help a student recognize that there are few absolutes in clinical work. Also, the supervisor must be willing to admit openly to a student when an error in judgment has been made. The supervisor must realize and bring the student to the realization that there will always be some wrong decisions and that they can be made by the most qualified, experienced clinicians (Schultz, 1972; 1975).

Even though many clinical decisions are perplexing, the supervisor need not be vague in articulating them to his student. Rather, the supervisor would be well advised to present himself and his ideas in such a way that they reflect self-confidence. This, in turn, should bolster the student's confidence in his supervisor. A student who is skeptical of his supervisor's capabilities cannot be expected to learn well if this attitude pervades his thinking. Under such circumstances, he may reject the supervisor's sound clinical decisions along with those that are seemingly unwise, an unfortunate consequence of the student's inability to tell the difference and/or his general condemnation of anything the supervisor attempts to teach. This potentially damaging situation can be averted by the actions and words of a poised, self-assured supervising clinician.

Experienced clinicians make fewer errors than do inexperienced clinicians. One deals more effectively with clinical problems if they are similar to previously encountered problems. Hence, the larger the repertoire of cases in a clinician's background, the better equipped he is to handle new challenges. Transferring this to the "master clinician" requirement for supervisory work, the logical conclusion is this: a supervisor should be an experienced clinician. This was recognized by Schubert in one of his suggested minimal requirements for supervisors, "two years of paid professional experience following the completion of the Clinical Fellowship Year" (1974, p. 305). This is equivalent to nearly three years' total experience beyond the graduate school training period, certainly not too stringent a requirement for supervisors in clinical audiology. Indeed, hindsight tells most audiologists who took on the job of clinical supervision immediately following graduation that they were not prepared for this work and that they learned as much as, or more than, their students did during those early years. Experience by no means ensures competence. Erroneous clinical thinking and faulty test procedures can be perpetuated for years. Fortunately, however, most dissatisfied patients and most unresolved clinical problems do not remain unnoticed forever. Such a natural accountability system plus the trial-and-error school of experience often serve as instructive vehicles for the clinician, helping him to develop and mature professionally.

To recapitulate, an effective supervisor is a competent and experienced clinician. Conversely, a competent, experienced clinician is not necessarily an effective supervisor. There are many additional prerequisites, some of which will now be considered.

Teaching Ability

Teaching ability constitutes the second major competency area and, as previously indicated, is one of Anderson's eight components of supervision (1973b, 1975). As also mentioned earlier, the teaching component will hereafter be regarded as the key competency, with Anderson's seven remaining components serving as integral parts thereof.

Supervision is teaching. Supervisors are teachers; that is, according to common dictionary definition, those who impart knowledge or skill, or who give instruction (Barnhart, 1968). To impart knowledge or skill successfully, one must be able to explain ideas clearly. This is the essence of clinical teaching. Lucid explanations or descriptions of clinical events and their rationale are of vital importance to the student's successful assimilation of classroom-learned facts. Although it is true that the clinical setting has its ready-made "audiovisual" aids (test equipment, test results, patients, and live action) to expedite the teaching/learning process, these same factors can just as easily contribute to the student's confusion. This happens most frequently when they interact in somewhat unpredictable ways, thus leaving the student in a quandary as he tries to reconcile clinical happenings that seem to conflict with his classroom/textbook learning. The supervisor is the only person who is in a position to bridge this gap, and it can be accomplished only through well-reasoned, logical explanations to the student. Furthermore, if the supervisor's interpretation of events is vague and/or inarticulate, he may succeed in baffling a student who had a better understanding of the material before the supervisor attempted to enlighten him.

To illustrate, the use of masking is frequently misunderstood by students. There are several reasons for this: (1) supervisors' misconceptions of masking principles and their clinical correlates, due to poor teaching of the supervisors themselves when they were students; (2) hazy explanations given by supervisors who perceive masking reasonably well but cannot translate their knowledge into understandable language; and (3) the variety of clinical procedures used in masking application. To counteract each of these potential obstacles, respectively, the audiology supervisor must acquire: (1) a firm understanding of masking; (2) a workable system of structured explanation in concrete, easily-understood terms; and (3) a set of masking procedures that is compatible with information given by course instructors and other supervisors within the same training program. With this kind of preparation, teaching effectiveness can be greatly enhanced at the clinical level.

Leadership Leadership is an important component of clinical teaching. Although it is ordinarily discussed in relation to group activities, leadership can, and does, apply to one-to-one teacher/student interactions, such as those found in clinically supervised audiology practicum. Inasmuch as the supervisor is guiding the student's pursuit of a set of definable goals or competencies, leadership is involved. Leadership has been thoroughly studied, and there is a body of literature devoted to exploring its intricacies. The following remarks will be limited to its connection with supervision in audiology.

To fulfill his capacity as teacher, the supervisor will necessarily find himself leading the student to perform a task that the supervisor has explained. In other words, the supervisor must induce the student to follow his guidance in a prescribed manner. Once the student has followed the supervisor's instruction, the supervisor then makes a judgment as to whether or not the student has complied satisfactorily. If performance has fallen short of the supervisor's expectations, he must act to rectify the situation. This entire leadership process needs to be handled tactfully by the supervisor if he wants to maintain a harmonious working relationship with the student, a relationship that will further the learning process rather than hinder it.[1]

Several pertinent, basic questions that an aspiring supervisor should be able to answer affirmatively are these: "Can I lead without being overbearing and autocratic? Can I help the student to see himself and me as a team working together to serve a patient? Can I give direction without being unduly demanding?" Thus, although the supervisor needs to assume authority, he must neither flaunt nor abuse it. Some suggested rules with illustrative dialogue follow.

> DO suggest, DON'T command: for example; "You might want to recheck those two thresholds," instead of "Those thresholds are wrong; recheck them."
>
> DO encourage self-discovery, DON'T always tell: for example; "Do you have the equipment set up right?" instead of "You set up the equipment wrong; I told you to use the right speaker, not the left speaker."
>
> DO give constructive criticism, DON'T give destructive criticism: for example; "You could have elaborated more on your explanation of lipreading to the patient," (followed by sample ideas that could have been included), instead of "Your explanation of lipreading to the patient was too brief," with no followup suggestions.
>
> DO balance negative comments with positive comments: for example; "Your description of test results in this report was good, but I made some changes in the paragraph dealing with our recommendations," followed by explanation of the corrections made.
>
> DO be firm, DON'T threaten: for example; "You've got to increase your speed in testing; there's just not enough time in a test session, nor should a patient be expected to withstand such a long ordeal," instead of "I don't think you're going to make it as a clinician unless you pick up a lot of speed, and soon."

Whenever corrections and/or advice are in order, the supervisor should use inoffensive words. The teaching/learning process will be well served if he tempers his remarks with a measure of kindness and respect for the student. If the student still finds it difficult to accept criticism (and many do), it behooves the supervisor to help the student understand that he is in a learning situation and therefore is not expected to be error-free at this stage in his career. On the other hand, there are those students who do need to be prodded into bettering their clinical performance. Although admonishment and appeal to reason may be called for, even these individuals will not be coaxed into self-motivation if the supervisor attempts to accomplish this through ridicule and insult. Such super-

---

[1] An excellent, practical treatise on the impact of human interaction in teacher-student relationships can be found in Gordon's T.E.T. Teacher Effectiveness Training (1974). A recent declaration of "Bills of Rights" for supervisors and supervisees in communicative disorders (Gerstman, 1977) is similarly applicable.

visory rebukes are generally counterproductive because they simply intimidate students. A student who is frightened or threatened by a supervisor's warning or ultimatum cannot be expected to perform optimally under such pressure. There are exceptions to this contention, but, in any case, the supervisor should carefully assess the situation before he adopts a "get tough" policy. Positive leadership is effective; negative leadership is risky.

By practicing positive, compassionate leadership, a supervisor can open the lines of communication between himself and his students. But these lines must be kept open by the supervisor through additional means, such as those discussed in the following comments on the teaching competency of communication.

Communication Because communication is a two-way process, it seems reasonable to propose that the supervisor not always be on the "giving end" and the student not always be on the "receiving end." In other words, the supervisor should allow the student ample opportunity to provide input through suggestions, questions, and general discussion (Pickering, 1977). This type of free-flowing communication serves several purposes: it lets the student know that the supervisor values his ideas, although the student may not fully realize this unless told; it allows the supervisor to examine from a different perspective the student's understanding of clinical information; and it gives the supervisor an opportunity to nurture the student's inquiring mind. In the matter of this last benefit of open communication, the supervisor must continually encourage each student to scrutinize all aspects of every case he sees and to question everything he does clinically. A cardinal rule should be set forth: that no single piece of clinical information ever be accepted at face value. That is to say, the student must learn to appreciate the importance of viewing information with a critical eye, and then balancing all factors with one another before he draws conclusions. This is vital to the production of thinking clinicians and is therefore to be cultivated in every aspiring clinical audiologist.

When the supervisor encounters a nonquestioning student who is reluctant to initiate discussion and/or verbalize ideas, he must make every attempt to elicit the student's thinking on matters at hand. If the reason for the student's self-imposed silence seems to be fear or shyness, it is the supervisor's responsibility to create a comfortable atmosphere that is conducive to honest, open discussion. There may be other reasons for a student's reticence; for example, he simply does not have enough knowledge to generate questions (unlikely but possible), or he has no sincere interest in the clinical assignment. Whatever the cause, the supervisor needs to ferret it out and deal with it accordingly. It is imperative that each student participate in clinical discussion. Such communication is an integral part of the clinical teaching/learning process.

Communication between supervisor and student is greatly affected by the supervisor's attitude, and consequently his behavior, toward the student. Indeed, the necessary comfortable atmosphere referred to in the preceding paragraph is largely dependent on the supervisor's disposition in the student's presence.[2] The supervisor's attitude is reflected in the ways he chooses to instruct or correct the student, as implied in the foregoing statements on teaching ability and leadership. However, there are a number of other ways in which he can disrupt communication lines between himself and the student. For example, he must not relate to a student with condescension. A patronizing attitude could easily be detected by a student under the following possible circumstances: the supervisor treats the student more as a child than as an adult; the supervisor embarrasses the student by pointing out the student's errors in the presence of a patient or others; the supervisor plays a game of one-upmanship with his student; the supervisor demands to be addressed formally instead of by his given name (acceptable, if not desirable, in front of the patients, but otherwise unnecessary[3]). Each of these behavioral displays is a sign that the supervisor is insecure in his roles as both clinician and supervisor. He can further impede communication by constantly interrupting a student who is trying to express an opinion or answer a question. If a student seldom has the chance to complete his statements, he will take the cue, whether it be intentional or unintentional on the supervisor's part, that his ideas are secondary in importance and that the supervisor is really not interested in his opinions.

The supervisor must pay heed to another important mode of expression, body language (Brown, 1975). He needs to be alert to his own facial expressions; for example, do they show approval or disapproval, pleasure or disgust? He needs to be aware of how he touches a student; for example, does he give the student an occasional reassuring pat on the back, or does he push the student aside in his eagerness to take the student's place in the test chair when the student is not performing satisfactorily? The supervisor also needs to sense other overt self-demonstrations of emotion; for example, is he tense and shaking, or calm and

---

[2] The student's attitude is also operative, as previously mentioned. This facet of the communicative link is not examined in the ensuing discussion, however, because the mission here is to consider desirable characteristics for the supervisor.

[3] Undoubtedly, many individuals in our field will disagree with this. But, in the author's opinion, use of Miss-Mrs.-Mr.-Doctor titles between student and supervisor promotes the inferior/superior attitudes associated with a hierarchy and needlessly creates a false barrier in the communication process. Competency, not titles, earns student respect.

relaxed? Does he pace the floor while the student is trying to complete a task, or does he stand by patiently? Does he sigh, groan, or otherwise show audible displeasure? Does he maintain eye contact with the student, and can he maintain this while he criticizes the student? These are but a few examples of the many ways in which a supervisor conveys messages without uttering a word. Obviously, the student does not need to be exceptionally perceptive in order to grasp their meaning. It is precisely because this form of communication is so powerful, yet so deceptively subtle, that a supervisor must be cognizant of his feelings and exert some control over them.

The supervisor's responsibilities in the promotion of fluid, productive communication are not confined to his relationship with the student, but must naturally be extended to the patient. This is clearly his duty as a clinician. However, beyond this, communicative skills with the patient must be first-rate because, as a supervisor, he is serving as a model for the student to emulate (as in the "master clinician" requirement). The supervisor model is unquestionably fundamental to clinical teaching, and it is within the area of clinician-patient intercommunication where this model becomes most instructive. This is quite likely the primary way in which students actually learn to communicate effectively with their patients. Although it is the supervisor's job to point out to the student reasonable approaches to communication with the patient, the example he sets in this regard will provide the more practical, hence better-remembered, set of initial learning experiences. Exemplary communication teaching takes place throughout the course of an audiologic evaluation in which the supervisor interacts with the patient, as evidenced by the following: the student observes how the supervisor talks to, looks at, and touches the patient; and he listens to the supervisor's reactions to the patient's comments, the kinds of questions the supervisor asks, and the ways in which the supervisor handles the patient's complaints. This unstructured form of teaching must always be taken into account by the supervisor, because it makes his communicative proficiency doubly important.

Interpersonal Relationships The category of interpersonal relationships is inextricably linked with the communication and leadership factors in supervision, because it is impossible to communicate or lead effectively in a one-to-one situation without a satisfactory interpersonal relationship. Nonetheless, the complexity of this area indicates the need for a more detailed consideration of its impact on audiology supervision.

When establishing interpersonal relationships, the supervisor needs to be extraordinarily flexible. Because a supervisor is the constant in a milieu of variables, it is he who must adapt to the ever-changing needs and personalities of students and patients. It is he who is primarily responsible for generating a climate of amicability between and among student, patient, and himself. And it is he who ultimately bears the burden of soothing the unhappy feelings of others, feelings of disappointment, guilt, dissatisfaction, fear, or animosity, whether they belong to patient or to student. This is a weighty responsibility, and it takes an emotionally mature person to handle it with sensitivity.

Although students have many characteristics and experiences in common, such as age, uncertainty about the future, and adjustment to the rigors of graduate school, they represent an infinite variety of dispositions. The supervisor needs to deal with their differences as well as their similarities. For example, at some time in his career, a supervisor is liable to encounter students having the following problems: inhibiting shyness; unabashed aggressiveness; underestimation or overestimation of their own knowledge and clinical potential; personality conflict with the supervisor; basic uncomfortableness in the clinical setting and/or the presence of the supervisor; or general dissatisfaction with the clinical assignment. These kinds of vexing problems must be confronted directly by the supervisor if he is at all conscientious about his obligations to troubled students. Through individual conferences, he and the student must attempt to solve the problem(s) together. This calls for frankness, openmindedness, and compromise on the part of both individuals.

Personality clashes between supervisor and student are probably the most difficult to resolve. Although the supervisor has every right to expect a student to be flexible in the relationship, it is incumbent upon the supervisor to be the more accommodating party, within reason. He must remember that it is his job to teach the student, to train him to be an effective clinician. If the attainment of that goal is served by humility and willingness to adapt one's mode of supervision, then so be it. To paraphrase a familiar quotation: if one is not part of the solution, one may be part of the problem. To see himself as part of the problem, to initiate acts of selflessness, to modify his supervision to suit each student's personality set—these are indications of a supervisor who has a healthy self-concept and can cope effectively with a host of student temperaments.

Although some supervisors appear to pursue the resolution of personal differences through student counseling with natural ease and apparent success, a background of courses in psychology, human relations, and counseling is an obvious asset. Even if the supervisor does not have professionally polished counseling skills, it is important that he have self-understanding and practical knowledge of human behavior before taking on the consequential responsibilities of student supervision.

Regardless of the preparatory steps taken, however, each supervisor will encounter students' personal problems that he cannot, and should not, attempt to solve. In such cases, it is hoped that he will recognize his limitations and refer the students for appropriate professional help (Pickering, 1977).

The subject of interpersonal relationships within the context of clinical supervision also embraces the patient. Given the gamut of individual personalities represented in a clinical population, it is not possible to detail them here. Suffice it to say that, although it is unlikely that the supervisor will become as personally involved with patients as he is with students, he must rely on his same resources of affability and flexibility. This constitutes partial fulfillment of the "master clinician" role, providing additional means whereby his communication model can be expanded for the student's sake. It is important for the student to observe the supervisor's maneuvering of clinician-patient-family interactions, especially those involving cantankerous or uncooperative patients and bickering patient/family situations. Moreover, the supervisor's attitude toward all kinds of patients should be shared openly with the student. It would be misleading, if not hypocritical, for the supervisor to disguise for the student any negative feelings he might harbor concerning certain patients. The student needs to know that the supervisor is emotionally responsive and that he, the student, is also entitled to have similar feelings. Self-righteousness has no place in the supervisor's character; if anyone is apt to detect phoniness, it is today's graduate student. But beyond this, the critical followup to any sharing of unpleasant feelings with the student is imperative. The supervisor must demonstrate to the student how he can transcend feelings and deal with patients effectively without alienating them.

Supervisors may not realize what a powerful impact their example-setting has on a student's thinking, particularly in the area of personal attitudes and interrelations. The student sees the supervisor not only as his teacher, but as a professional, on-the-job audiologist, someone to emulate if the student respects the supervisor's thinking. The supervisor's opinions of his own work, of audiology as a field, of associated otologists, hearing aid dealers and agencies, as well as his posture on patient management, will combine to formulate or greatly affect the eventual attitudes and actions of impressionable students. Such potential influence on future audiologists, and thus the field, carries with it a great responsibility that should never be taken lightly.

Analysis and Facilitation   Analysis and facilitation, the next clinical teaching factors to be examined, are part of an ongoing process for the supervisor in audiology. Analysis involves those considerations that form the substance of clinical decision making, while facilitation connotes the accommodating actions based on these decisions.

The supervisor must be able to analyze the situation before him at any given moment, and then make appropriate clinical and supervisory decisions. In a developing test session, the options may change from minute to minute, thereby forcing quick decisions. By contrast, analysis of student performance over time, for example, week by week, can be based on an evolving series of observations and decisions. Some varied samples of analytical thinking typically faced by a supervisor are represented by the following questions he might ask himself: "Does this student appear to be ready to counsel the type of patient we are evaluating this morning? Did the student perform poorly today because he was worried about his midterm exam, or am I beginning to see a regression in his clinical performance? Does this patient seem to be bothered by the fact that a student is working with him? Is there time to give the student a detailed explanation of our recommendations; or should it be done after the patient is gone; or should it not be done at all in order to ascertain if the student has been observant and perceptive, reaching conclusions on his own? Why is this student having so much difficulty grasping the concept of overmasking?" The interplay of patient, student, and supervisor with one another and with factors of time and circumstance, sets the course for supervisory option analysis.

Facilitation, the expediting action based on careful analysis, quite often pertains to the actual balancing of a patient's needs with a student's needs, so that each individual derives optimal benefit while, at the same time, the audiologic session proceeds smoothly. This facilitation of the simultaneous operations of student training and patient service can be an exceedingly complicated maneuver for the supervisor, particularly if the setting is an active, fast-paced clinic. Because of the conflicting time demands made by patient vs. student, the analysis stage must first culminate in the supervisor's establishing of priorities, and then in compromise. The ensuing facilitation process demands manipulation of people and situations in concert. Although the supervisor's judgment should be based on immediate assessment of each set of circumstances, there is a basic philosophical issue to be considered: to whom is the supervisor more duty-bound, the patient or the student? The easy answer is that he has an equal obligation to both. In reality, this answer often does not translate into a practical solution. A choice must be made.

Having experienced many agonizing decisions over this dilemma, it is my considered opinion that patient service comes before student training in any situation where *all* feasible alternatives have been ruled out. This does not mean, however, that student learning need be sacrificed. In the first place, when such a conflict arises, the supervisor should inform the student of his plans and the rationale behind any decision to accommodate the patient. This very discussion, and the reasoning that prompted it, should be instructive for the student. Secondly, the student is still in a position to learn from whatever is transpiring, whether he is asked to observe temporarily while the supervisor takes over, or required to perform a task without accompanying detailed explanation by the supervisor. In either instance, the supervisor can supplement his instruction during a postsession conference with the student. Not incidentally, this is another step in the continuing task of facilitation.

Just as facilitation for the patient's sake should not diminish a supervisor's commitment to any student, compromise on the student's behalf does not release the supervisor from his obligations to clinical service. (Yet the latter condition exists during every moment of ongoing student instruction while the patient is present.) The supervisor must recognize that he cannot be everything to both parties at all times. The key to successful facilitation lies in his ability to balance the needs of student and patient over several hours' time. For example, if a prepared student is asked to relinquish his counseling opportunity for the first patient in a half-day assignment, the supervisor should make every attempt to ensure that the student does not miss participation in that same activity with the next patient. By the same token, if said second patient appears to be understanding and tolerant, the supervisor might choose to give additional detailed hearing aid instruction to the student while the patient is present. And so the bartering goes in both directions.

There is quite another form of facilitation in supervised audiology practicum. It calls for resourcefulness on the part of the supervisor, and it involves coordination of his leadership, communication, and personal relationship competencies. It is this: a supervisor should make use of his capacity to exert a positive influence on any unproductive or self-defeating traits that are manifested clinically by students or patients. He can draw on the aforementioned competencies to motivate others to change their attitudes and behavior in a positive direction. As practiced in psychological counseling and group leadership circles, this mode of facilitation implies the reinforcement of one stimulus by another stimulus. In the context of audiology supervision, stimulus/stimulus reinforcement can be accomplished directly by the supervisor with either his patient or his student. More indirect methods are also workable, as in the case of a supervisor's inducing the student to influence a patient or, perhaps, a situation in which the supervisor elicits self-behavior modification in the patient or the student. Regardless of the approach, the supervisor is the primary facilitator, the instigator.

Because he is not a professional psychologist or a trained group facilitator, the audiology supervisor must be careful not to overstep his bounds. But he does have an obligation to further the goals of his patients (improved communicative efficiency) and his students (increased clinical competence) through every possible means. For instance, a student may be stimulated to become more responsive or more conscientious in his clinical work, or a patient might be moved to accept his hearing loss more realistically or change his attitude toward hearing aid use. Because the supervisor has more frequent, intimate contact with students than with patients, such efforts are likely to be more effective with the students; and where the opportunity is greater, so is the responsibility greater. The one-to-one teacher/student bond in a regularly scheduled clinical activity creates an ideal environment for methodical behavior shaping. In the interest of student growth, the supervisor should capitalize on this special opportunity afforded by clinical teaching. If he facilitates with skill, he can bring out the best in his students.

Management   Supervision in a university training program encompasses four distinct areas of management: patient, student clinician, clinic, and academic. The peculiarities of one's job govern the amount of time and energy devoted to each area.

Skillful, innovative patient management is an obvious ingredient of the "master clinician" specification. It includes management of the patient while he is in the clinical environment, making appropriate recommendations and referrals, following the patient's progress, and maintaining contact with the involved outside sources (otologist, hearing aid dealer, agency) to exchange information. That portion of patient management that is conducted in the joint presence of student and patient can readily be demonstrated and/or explained to the student. However, the supervisor needs to make a special effort to keep students informed of followup management activities. Too often, audiology students see patients only for the first step of a multi-appointment sequence; hence, they do not know the eventual outcome of their initial clinical efforts. Such incomplete clinical teaching can be minimized by an alert supervisor.

Management of the student clinician takes in all of the supervisor/ student interrelations heretofore discussed. Bearing in mind the number and difficulty of these supervisory tasks, one comes to the logical, and perhaps ultimate, question that every aspiring supervisor needs to ask himself: "Do I want the dual responsibility of managing both a student and a patient at the same time?" If the answer is negative, supervision should clearly not be pursued. If the answer is uncertain or affirmative, supervision practicum is in order, as discussed in Chapter 5.

Both clinic management and academic involvement can take on significant importance in the university supervisor's total role, especially if they consume a substantial amount of time and energy. Clinic management, for example, can include such duties as determining both patient appointment and overall time schedules, maintaining a hearing aid inventory, and promoting professional liaisons. Management of academic obligations often entails the scheduling of students' clinical practicum assignments, faculty/staff meetings, inservice training programs, and simply keeping abreast of curriculum developments within the training program. All such activities can serve the supervisor's teaching facility. In fact, he should seize every possible opportunity to share germane information (for example, new hearing aids in stock) with his students. The inclusion of students in discussion of daily clinic happenings not only adds measurably to their learning about the field of audiology, but it gives them a more involved, more important feeling about their status as student clinicians.

Evaluation   The final competency in the teaching ability category is evaluation. Because this plays such an important role in clinical supervision, it is clear that the effective supervisor must be a proficient evaluator of students' clinical performance. Unlike the periodic tests given in a classroom to evaluate students' knowledge of specific subjects, clinical evaluation is an ongoing process, one that enables the supervisor to choose and change his levels of supervision for each student. Clinical evaluation must probe areas other than *knowledge,* that is, the student's understanding of audiologic concepts. It also needs to examine: (1) a student's clinical *knowhow,* or, his ability to integrate knowledge, and then apply it clinically; (2) his clinical *insight,* or, his capacity to see the patient as a person and make decisions accordingly; and (3) his clinical *personality,* or, how he relates to patients and how he responds to the supervisor's instruction. Because these latter competency areas are more intangible than classroom-measured knowledge, they are more difficult to quantify and their evaluation is largely subjective. Furthermore, the evaluator must look at all areas repeatedly, taking into account a student's long-term memory capacity as well as his ability to learn from self-discovered and supervisor-corrected errors. Clinical evaluation is therefore complex, but it does serve several purposes in clinical teaching. Following are examples of how a supervisor might use evaluation to determine his teaching approach in masking, vis-a-vis four competency areas.

Clinical Knowledge   A student does not fully understand basic masking principles. He may need some individual tutoring from the supervisor outside clinic hours, and/or the supervisor might send the student home with sample audiograms to study. In any event, more supervisory time per patient will need to be devoted to this student.

Clinical Knowhow   A student understands basic masking principles and, in fact, can discuss them in depth. However, when faced with a patient whose hearing loss requires the use of masking, the student becomes confused and performs as though he has no understanding of masking. The supervisor must determine the reason for this apparent discrepancy, and then act accordingly. Some of the techniques as cited in the clinical knowledge area may be indicated, along with step-by-step supervisory instruction during actual testing. Postevaluation discussion of those cases which proved troublesome is especially important.

Clinical Insight   A student understands masking principles and ordinarily can administer tests requiring the use of masking. However, when faced with a patient who does not comprehend the listening task required of him and therefore responds inappropriately, the student does not recognize the problem or is unable to solve it. The supervisor must call this situation to the student's attention, give him sample solutions (reinstructing the patient, varying stimuli presentation, using a more expedient masking technique), then help the student to attack the problem. Postevaluation discussion is essential, and close supervision of future similar cases may be indicated.

Clinical Personality   A student seems to conduct masking procedures ineptly under close supervision, but apparently does a better job when the supervisor is situated in an adjacent room. The only reasonable supervisory approach is to vary the near and far placements so the student can be monitored regularly, yet without constant vigilance. A chat with the student about his uncomfortableness in the supervisor's presence is also indicated.

Not only does evaluative identification of student strengths and weaknesses help the supervisor to modify instruction, but it aids the student directly, if the supervisor keeps him informed as to his progress. Furthermore, the results of clinical evaluation can be used to monitor a student's progress from term to term in his total practicum sequence, so that: appropriate clinical assignments can be made in subsequent terms; supervisors can know in advance what a student's specific needs are; letters of recommendation can eventually be written; and decisions regarding a future in clinical audiology can be reached for those students receiving consistently poor evaluations from various supervisors.

The final, and quite likely the most controversial, aspect of clinical evaluation is the resultant letter grade. Given the present system of quantifying academic achievement within a university, clinical performance warrants credit hours and grades and assigned teachers just as do the classroom courses. When transcripts for students are forwarded to prospective employers, the applicant's clinical grades may carry considerable weight. Evaluation is thus a key component of the clinical teaching process. (Details of evaluation procedures are discussed in the next chapter.)

QUALITIES

Because all of the supervisory competencies have been presented as outlined at the beginning of this discussion, what follows is a briefer consideration of desirable supervisor qualities.

Patience

The first desirable quality is patience. Unless a person has a great deal of patience, all thoughts of clinical supervision should seriously be reconsidered. Examples of the types of patience required in an audiology supervisor include: tolerance of others' errors, even when repeated continually; tolerance of relatively slow learners; perseverance in explaining and re-explaining, and in reminding and reviewing; indefatigability in working with new classes of beginners year after year; and diligence in providing each student with as much clinical expertise as time and capacity will allow within a given assignment. Because it is recognized that one needs to have an ample supply of patience in order to be a competent clinical audiologist in the first place, these additional exacting demands create a niche for a special kind of person. Not every audiologist has the temperament for this type of work. It is precisely at those moments when a supervisor runs out of patience that quality supervision is compromised, for it is during these times that he becomes irritated, unnecessarily takes over the student's work, minimizes detailed instruction, or otherwise shirks the responsibilities of supervision.

Sense of Humor

A responsive sense of humor is a welcome supervisor quality. Three parties stand to benefit from this attribute—the supervisor, the student, and the patient. Certainly, the supervisor needs it to sustain himself. And, although it is important that he take his job seriously, it is also the supervisor's duty to create a relaxed atmosphere for the student. This can be accomplished largely through the sharing of humorous moments. Most students respond in kind, thereby keeping lines of communication open. Furthermore, the supervisor must be willing to laugh at his own mistakes, freely admitting such errors to the student. This strengthens the supervisor/student relationship, in that the student gains respect for his supervisor's honesty while learning that mistakes are acceptable and, if admitted and corrected, harmless. Finally, the expression of humor to patients, when done tastefully and at the appropriate time, helps to reduce any tension in the test situation. This, also, is part of the supervisor's modeling for the student.

Commitment to Clinical Supervision

Another noteworthy quality that should be required of the potential audiology supervisor is sincere commitment to clinical supervision. Although it might seem apparent that all clinical supervisors aspire to their roles, such is not the case. Many are clinical audiologists who were given the added responsibilities of student supervision after they began employment. Others may have sought supervisory posts because they thought their workloads would be lightened with the help of a student assistant. Most supervisors in either of these groups care little about clinical teaching, and student learning is likely to suffer. If, by implicit actions or attitude, a supervisor lets a student know that he is a brake to a normally efficient operation or, conversely, that he is the supervisor's assistant and thereby expected to undertake a major portion of the workload, unsupervised, the student will surely be quick to perceive the situation.

Interest in Continued Learning

An audiology supervisor must demonstrate interest in his own continued learning. He not only needs to show enthusiasm about each patient seen, but he should convey to the student a sense of intellectual curiosity about unresolved clinical questions. The supervisor can further inspire a student by discussing with him current developments in the field as they relate to mutual clinical cases. Moreover, it is incumbent upon the person responsible for clinical teaching to stay well informed, because the field is changing and expanding so rapidly. And the supervisor's quest for new ideas need not be limited to rhetoric. Insofar as possible, supervisors should engage in clinical experimentation.

CONCLUSION

The foregoing discussion covers important factors that contribute to successful clinical supervision. The two basic competencies, clinical skill and teaching skill, shape the foundation. But teaching practicum cannot be effective unless it includes competence in such areas as leadership, communication, interpersonal relationships, analysis, facilitation, management, and evaluation. In addition, a supervisor's effectiveness will be enhanced by certain qualities, including patience, sense of humor, commitment to clinical supervision, and interest in continued learning in the profession. All contribute to good supervision. Good supervision will not materialize, however, without a workable supervisory strategy, such as the one proposed in the next chapter.

CHAPTER 4

A BASIC MODEL OF SUPERVISION IN AUDIOLOGY

CONTENTS

In accordance with the notion that there are as many definitions and conceptions of the clinical supervisor and the supervision process in audiology as there are persons involved in supervision, one can carry the premise a step further: there are as many variations in actual methodology as there are individuals fulfilling supervisory roles in audiology. This state of affairs is clearly traceable to the dearth of uniform preparation for audiology supervision, as discussed in the introductory chapter. And it is underscored by the reports of students who have participated in clinical practicum under the supervision of various persons, whether from different training programs or from within the same program. That there are such individual differences is not necessarily undesirable, of course, because a student's clinical learning experiences can be enriched considerably via exposure to various supervising clinicians. However, students also report that their various supervised experiences have differed in quality; that is to say, they "learned more" from some supervisors than they did from others. Although these judgments sometimes reflect individual student/supervisor personality conflicts and/or the diversity of clinical settings (hence, different patient populations) in which the students gained their practicum experiences, it is equally tenable to attribute such remarks to disparities in supervisory technique.

Given these assertions, there is a need to subject the currently used methods of supervision in audiology to close scrutiny, to determine why some of them are apparently effective and others are not, and then to discard the unworkable ideas and disseminate those that have proven their worth. In view of the absence of such precedents, as well as the lack of controlled research efforts in this area, a basic model of supervision in audiology is presented in this chapter for the readers' consideration. Lest a detailed presentation of this kind seem presumptuous on the part of the author, such is not the intent. Rather, I am hopeful that other audiology supervisors will relate these ideas to their own efforts and, in so doing, find reason to disclose tested methods of their own. The resultant dialogue may then generate some research investigations into the validity of certain techniques and the development of new ones. The objective is evident: improved supervision in audiology.

Because procedural matters are partly determined by the nature of the clinic and the university training program in which a supervisor functions, a general description of the Northwestern University modus operandi is in order. Students seeking a master's degree in audiology are normally placed in a two year (seven quarter) combined sequence of courses and clinical assignments. As a rule, the latter spans six of the seven quarters because most new students are not given clinical practicum assignments during their first quarter in graduate school; exceptions are made for those students having a particularly strong undergraduate background in speech and hearing, if the clinical assignment schedule can accommodate them. Preprofessional students whose audiology coursework was initiated during their senior year at Northwestern University are also enrolled in the clinical practicum sequence at an earlier stage. The usual coursework schedule is completed by the end of six quarters to enable all students to participate in advanced, externship clinical assignments, primarily in off-campus settings, on a fulltime basis during their last quarter preceding graduation. Although the five to six quarters of "regular" clinical practicum are conducted primarily in the on-campus clinical sites on the Evanston and Chicago (medical school) campuses by university supervisory personnel, more off-campus facilities, such as hospitals, public health stations and school-affiliated clinics, have been utilized in recent years due to the increasing demands of an extended clinical training program. Assignments are allotted in half-day blocks of time, and the supervisor-to-student ratio for any given assignment is one-to-one to allow for individualized clinical teaching. Each student is required to register in a clinical study course at the beginning of every school quarter in order to become eligible for clinical assignments; thus he receives a grade and university credit for his clinical practicum work. In addition, all such registrants must participate in a weekly two-hour seminar that is designed to supplement the practicum training through coverage of a wide variety of clinical topics. These seminars are coordinated by an academic faculty person, but include active participation by other clinical supervisors and invited speakers.

A meeting of staff supervisors is held prior to the beginning of each school quarter for the purpose of scheduling students for their clinical assignments. Inasmuch as most audiology courses are, by design, offered in the afternoon to facilitate the scheduling process, clinical assignments can be scheduled primarily through the morning and noon hours. Nonetheless, the task is not easily accomplished, given the many factors that need to be taken into consideration: for example, conflicting time slots of elective courses; distance of satellite clinical facilities from campus; and students' preference, or readiness, for certain assignments. The student readiness factor causes an exceedingly difficult scheduling problem, in that all students should ideally be assigned first to clinical practica involving fundamental clinical competencies (for example, basic audiometric testing for adults), and then progress to assignments requiring more advanced skills (pediatric audiology, hearing aid selection, special auditory testing). As stated in Chapter 2, orderly competency building, although desirable, can only be achieved to a certain degree. This holds true in the scheduling process also, because it is impossible to tailor clinic schedules to meet precisely the needs of a structured student training program. Yet, an attempt is made to meet these needs in several ways. As is undoubtedly the case in most training programs, clinically related courses are sequenced in order of complexity; for example, the hearing measurements course precedes the amplification course, which precedes the special auditory testing courses, and so on. In like manner, the clinical seminar topics are grouped in order of increasing sophistication. And, finally, the on-campus clinic schedules are controlled in such a way that students can be assigned to certain exclusive types of clinical participation, such as basic audiometric testing for adults, hearing aid selection for adults, and so forth. Indeed, some of the supervisory work has been compartmentalized so that several supervisors can devote themselves to working only with adults, only with children, or only in the diagnostic special test unit. Thus, the students' schedules are somewhat conformable to an orderly sequence; even so, simple logistics preclude ideal scheduling for each student every quarter. This forces the staff to stagger the assignments as equitably as possible.

A student is typically given two or three weekly half-day assignments per quarter, thereby affording him the opportunity to work with several different supervisors and in more than one clinical setting each quarter. He thus can accumulate eight to 12 clinical clock hours per week during the majority of his five to six quarters' "regular" assignments, and then another nine weeks' fulltime clinical experience during the aforementioned externship period. Most students, then, have in excess of 500 clinical clock hours by the time they graduate. And they acquire this practicum experience in at least four or five clinical settings under the guidance of just as many, or more, different supervisors. Conversely, this means that a given on-campus supervisor typically works with four to six different students per week, and he may encounter any student again in a subsequent quarterly clinical assignment. Thus, a supervisor may very well work with a student during his initial clinical work, and then again when that student is functioning at a more advanced level.

The supervision model that is presented in the following pages is a direct outgrowth of my participation in the clinical training program just described. However, the ideas do not necessarily reflect the opinions or supervisory techniques of my coworkers, nor do they represent official policy of the Northwestern University audiology program. Instead, these ideas are based on my personal views of audiology supervision, views which developed over more than a decade through the trial-and-error system of learning to supervise. Although the methods presented here seem to work reasonably well in my own particular job of supervising students in a medical school setting while working with an adult-only population,[1] the experimenting continues. Today's methods might not work with tomorrow's student. Be that as it may, they may provide guidelines for the beginning supervisor and food for thought to the experienced supervisor. In the interest of those who might wish to use this material as a sort of reference manual, a combined outline-expository format is used; some items necessarily contain ideas already mentioned in earlier chapters.

I. Clinic orientation   When a supervisor and a student meet each other for the first time under the circumstances in which they will be working together, certain preparatory activities are required. The supervisor needs to set aside some time for this orientation period, either by arranging to meet with the student on a day prior to the first day of actual clinical work, or by reducing the patient load on that first day

---

[1] The fact that these supervisory experiences grew out of clinical work with adults exclusively should be kept in mind throughout one's reading of this chapter. In many instances, of course, the supervisory approach may be identical regardless of the age range of the clinical population, but there are obvious points of divergence. Likewise, it should be noted that none of the ensuing methodology will include supervision of clinical practicum involving special auditory test batteries. Regardless, an overall pattern and its applicability in many areas of audiology instruction will become apparent to the reader.

A. Get acquainted with the student to "break the ice"; make him feel comfortable
   1. Discuss his background: previous clinical assignments, undergraduate preparation
   2. Ask how he became interested in the field of audiology
B. Explain clinical assignment to him:
   1. Types of patients, appointments, time allotments
   2. Individual approach to supervision, for example:
      a. How closely student will be supervised, and how this is determined
      b. Use of supervisor/student team approach
      c. Goals of supervisor *and* student for the ensuing quarter of clinical practicum
C. Apprise student of his clinical surroundings:
   1. Where patient records are kept
   2. Where to hang coat, keep personal belongings; location of bathroom, lunchroom facilities
   3. Introduction to coworkers: secretary, receptionist, and other staff members
D. Familiarize student with test facilities:
   1. Demonstrate equipment to be used:
      a. When, where to turn on, off
      b. How to operate: pure tone audiometer, speech audiometer, narrow band masker, otoadmittance meter, and any other instruments likely to be put into use for a particular assignment. When demonstrating equipment, the *rationale* behind every control manipulation should be explained carefully; the better the student understands instrumentation, the more easily he will remember operation procedures
      c. Tapes to be used: how to thread on recorder, how to set calibration tone, and the underlying rationale for these steps
   2. Review hearing aid stock and accessories:
      a. Hearing aid summary chart, manual, and manufacturers' specification sheets
      b. Hearing aids in stock
      c. Earmolds, tubing
      d. Tools, stethoscope
      e. Batteries, battery tester
   3. Show test room, counseling and patient waiting areas:
      a. Where patient, family members sit

b.   Location of response signals, earphones, bone conduction oscillator

4.   Review test forms and patient record forms to be used

II.   Listening check of equipment   Because daily listening checks of
test equipment are necessary, the student should be required to
participate in this important procedure before each clinical practicum session with the supervisor

A.   Discuss purpose of listening check

B.   Demonstrate steps of listening check, explaining why each
one is carried out; for example, clarity of signal, linearity of
signal, attenuator or other line noise, equipment hookup. This
demonstration/discussion can take place while the student
listens, with the supervisor telling the student what to listen
for

C.   After several sessions of having the student listen as the
supervisor operates equipment, reverse the procedure; advise
accordingly

D.   Once the student has mastered both "ends" of the listening
check, reverse roles from time to time

E.   Although listening checks in a two-room test suite can be
more easily accomplished by two persons, and the supervisor
can use this situation as a teaching vehicle, he should also
show the student how to conduct a rudimentary check of test
equipment on his own to prepare the student for times when a
second listener is not available

F.   Because the goal of biological equipment checks is trouble-
shooting, it is sometimes instructive for the supervisor to
"create" an equipment problem; this may often be the only
way in which one can find out what the student's detective
capabilities are, and whether or not he knows how to handle
minor equipment problems after he has isolated them

III.   Review of medical records and other patient information

A.   Before the arrival of each patient, review all available,
pertinent information step by step with the student, discussing
its implications for testing. The advanced student should do
this on his own, then discuss with supervisor. The supervisor,
in turn, should ask questions to determine if the student has
appropriately integrated the material, understands its
potential implications, and knows how to proceed

B.   Help the student to incorporate already-known information
into the patient's history record. Discuss. The student should
eventually be required to do this without assistance

IV. Patient interview
   A. Preparation for interview
      1. This step follows naturally from III. On the basis of depth, scope, and estimated accuracy of available information, decide with student which areas need to be explored further, which ones can be checked for confirmation, and which ones omitted from the interview
      2. Prestructure as deemed necessary
      3. If something unusual is known about the patient beforehand that might affect the interview approach, this should be discussed
   B. Interview
      1. For new students, the interview should be conducted by the supervisor during the first few sessions to provide a model. As the student listens and observes, he should have in hand a history form to follow. For the advanced student who has never before worked with the current supervisor, the supervisor's model interview can be limited to one session
         a. As the student listens and observes, it may be instructive to have him record information on his form at the same time the supervisor is doing so while interviewing the patient. Comparisons can then be made later, giving the supervisor an opportunity to discuss appropriate recording methods, terminology, and other pertinent aspects of the interview
         b. With some patients, at the supervisor's discretion, it is possible to take time, between questions of the patient, to explain to the student the rationale for a particular action (for example, why a question was phrased a certain way, or the reason behind probing for additional information in a specific area), or what is planned next, and the reasons for this decision
      2. As soon as the supervisor feels that the student has been exposed to enough sample interviews, the student should be asked to do them. (Prestructuring will probably be required for a period of time, however, until the student has gained some interview experience, with resultant insight into the process)
         a. Supervisor should listen in control room or adjacent room via intercom, making mental or written notes on student's performance

       b. If deemed necessary and/or appropriate, supervisor may intervene to assist student or give him suggestions; but consideration must first be given as to whether or not this will actually help the student and whether or not the patient will mind

       c. Another way to deal with incorrectly phrased or unasked questions is to review them with the student after the interview, then have him complete the task with his patient. This sometimes has negative consequences when a skeptical patient realizes that the student clinician has just consulted with his supervisor. If additional questions are not complicated, this potential conflict can be circumvented by having the student obtain the needed information from the patient when he returns to the test room for other reasons (e.g., to replace earphones with bone conduction oscillator), and does not have the history form in hand

  C. Postinterview discussion

    1. Briefly (for the patient's sake) review with the student his interview performance, pointing out strengths and weaknesses, asking for more information as noted in IV, B, 2, c, and discussing implications of patient information for test purposes

    2. Check student's written history and discuss strengths and weaknesses therein, making comments and suggestions, and adding or changing information on form when necessary

    3. If patient information is obtained at any time during the remainder of the audiologic evaluation, add to form and discuss with student

V. Test instructions

  A. Preparation

    1. For each new set of test instructions never before given by the student (e.g., air conduction pure tone, bone conduction pure tone, speech reception threshold, speech discrimination, masking, hearing aid tests), the supervisor should give at least one sample to a patient as the student listens

    2. Until the student has demonstrated complete independence in giving concise, flexible, clear instructions, the supervisor can prepare him by:

       a. Telling him exactly what to say

        b.   Having him give sample instructions to the super-visor as supervisor assumes role of patient

        c.   Giving him alternative approaches, pointing out the strong and weak points of each

    3.   Beware of transforming the student into a robot who gives a set of memorized instructions without thinking about what he is saying to the patient

    4.   Explain the importance of helping the patient to *understand* what is happening. As an example, in sound field speech reception threshold measurements, unaided and aided, the instructions can be supplemented with an explanation to the patient that the clinicians are trying to determine the softest level at which he can understand the words, first without a hearing aid, then with a hearing aid

    5.   Discuss the importance of adapting instruction terminology to patients' levels of understanding

  B. Instructions

    1.   If the supervisor gives instructions, he should be sure that the student understands why he is saying what he is saying

    2.   If the student gives instructions, the supervisor can listen from an adjacent room. If the supervisor is in the test room with the patient and student to observe subsequent earphone placement (as would be done with a beginning student), the supervisor can monitor the instructions while there, and then make appropriate suggestions to the student immediately, or add to his instructions if it is determined that the patient is confused and the student is lost

  C. Postinstruction discussion

    1.   Discuss with the student what was right, and what was wrong, with instructions, regardless of who gave them

    2.   Discuss whether or not the patient seemed to understand the instructions, and why or why not. Point out that a patient may not always understand what he is to do even if the instructions were well stated

VI. Earphone, bone conduction oscillator placement

  A. Demonstrate proper earphone, bone conduction oscillator placement several times, explaining to the student the reason for each step

  B. After the demonstrations, have the student perform this activity, commenting and assisting as necessary

  C. Thereafter, periodically check patients to determine if

student's positioning of earphones, oscillator is correct. The supervisor may be surprised to find out how often faulty placement is the cause of a test problem, for example, bone conduction oscillator touching pinna, or opposite phone slipping backwards and occluding ear canal during bone conduction masking

D. Always look through window between control room and test room to check on right vs. left earphone placement, masking phone position, and whether or not the bone conduction oscillator is on the correct mastoid. Such supervisory vigilance is indicated for even the more advanced students, as it allows detection of errors before they cause testing problems and waste time needlessly; the student need not know that the supervisor is checking this every time

VII. Pure tone audiometry, masking[2]

A. Discuss in detail the rationale for each and every step in testing until the student reaches the point at which he can explain to the supervisor what he is doing, why he is doing it, and whether or not the results seem credible

B. For the beginner, the supervisor should demonstrate the administration of each test several times so that the student can see how it is done before he attempts to do it himself. The supervisor needs to discuss each step as it is carried out. The student's experiences at this point will differ greatly from those he had when testing his classmates' hearing or working on a simulator for class projects, as he observes the handling of inconsistent responders, false-positive responders, and other difficult-to-test patients

C. As the student begins to participate in actual testing, the supervisor should sit alongside the student, watching each step and "thinking aloud" for the student until he gains some independence. This close watch is important, for example, during pure tone masking procedures, because the supervisor cannot look at a final masking amount and know how the

---

[2] To underscore the importance of effective supervision in this area, consider Jerger's words: "The assumption that comparatively low-level technicians can be quickly trained to carry out basic audiometry is one of the great myths of our time. It should not go unchallenged. One of the first lessons the observant clinical supervisor learns is that obtaining a seemingly simple pure tone audiogram often requires a considerable degree of prior training and insight. . . . People who trust the audiograms of minimally trained personnel have not yet learned how terribly wrong they can be in all but mild to moderate, bilaterally symmetrical, sensorineural loss." (1974, p. 249).

student derived it and whether or not his final results are valid, unless he actually taps the student's thinking process and sees how he operates the equipment throughout this procedure

D. Explain, illustrate recording procedures: symbols, masking levels, explanatory notes, test reliability comments

E. Gradually depart from close surveillance, step by step, as the student demonstrates proficiency through his own initiative

    1. Pull away from tasks in order of difficulty, e.g., air conduction first, bone conduction second, and so on, as in the skill competency scales, if reasonable

    2. Continue to spot check all tasks from time to time to analyze the situation. For example:

        a. Is student obtaining thresholds in the anticipated range?

        b. How consistent are the patient's responses?

        c. Is the better ear being tested first?

        d. Is the student taking an inordinate amount of time?

F. When not watching the student closely on each task, monitor from adjacent room to determine whether or not the student seems to be progressing satisfactorily. Through "listening," an alert supervisor can detect such problems as erroneous equipment setup, lapses in clear instruction-giving, as well as apparently unjustifiable slowness in the student's testing

G. For difficult-to-test patients (for example, inconsistent responder, bilateral conductive hearing loss with overmasking risks), the student may need to be closely supervised even though he has proven that he can perform these same tasks independently on more straightforward cases

H. Regardless of how advanced the student is in these areas, he should be required to show the supervisor his test results at certain points during the evaluation. This can be done, for example, when air conduction testing is completed, then when bone conduction thresholds have been obtained for the better ear, and so on. At each juncture, ask what he plans to do next and his reasons, until this is no longer deemed necessary. But still continue to review his test results at these points

I. With regard to pure tone masking procedures: if the supervisor has not been watching the student closely during the masking process and the final results, in the supervisor's judgment, do not appear credible, then it may be necessary to ask the student to recheck a threshold or two in the supervisor's presence. In this way, one can see firsthand how the patient's thresholds shifted or did not shift, whether or not the masking unit was turned on correctly, if the patient needs to be reinstructed, and the like. Of course, if the supervisor discovers, on this recheck, that the student was in error, close watch of this particular task should be resumed during testing of the next case. (A cardinal rule for all masking instruction is: repeat, repeat, repeat, repeat)

VIII.   Speech audiometry
    A.   As in other areas, discuss in detail the rationale for each step until the student reaches the point at which he can explain what he is doing, why he is doing it, and whether or not the results seem logical to him
    B.   For the beginner, demonstrate each task (speech reception threshold, discrimination testing, speech awareness threshold—via tape or monitored live voice) at least once before asking the student to do it. As the supervisor is performing each task, the student should be given a step-by-step explanation
    C.   Then observe as student performs each task, making appropriate comments and suggestions. Before each task is begun, discuss with student what he plans to do. Sample preparatory decisions might be:
        1.   Which ear should be tested first?
        2.   What is a reasonable beginning presentation level?
        3.   When familiarizing the patient with spondees, what should be done about the words that he misses:
            a.   Eliminate from list, but use tape?
            b.   Eliminate from list, but use monitored live voice?
            c.   Familiarize at higher level, lower level?
            d.   Change spondee material?
        4.   What presentation levels should be used for discrimination testing, and why?
        5.   Will masking be needed? If so, how much, and why?
        6.   How is equipment to be set up?
    For some time, it will be necessary for the supervisor to initiate these questions and to go through the thinking process with the student. Gradually, the clue-giving should be stopped and the student should be asked what he plans to do and what the reasons are behind his decisions, until he reaches the point at which he can make sound judgments without preliminary

discussion. At this stage, the supervisor can spot check the equipment settings to determine if the student's decisions are reasonable, then ask him questions to ascertain what his thinking process was. (Beware of the student who may happen to use a reasonable presentation level or the correct amount of masking, yet does now know why he made a particular choice)

D. During the actual testing procedure, gradually withdraw from the close-watch stance as the student acquires independence on each task, but again:

1. Continue to spot check, less frequently as time goes by, to be sure equipment is set up correctly

2. Monitor the student from an adjacent room even when not watching him closely. This can be accomplished easily during speech audiometry procedures if the loudspeaker of the talkback system is turned on. For example, the supervisor:

a. Can usually tell immediately if student is obtaining other-than-expected results

b. Can tell if patient understands the task

c. Can usually tell if student has failed to introduce masking

d. Can hear patient's responses

Throughout all monitoring of test procedures in this manner, including pure tone testing and masking as noted in VII, E, the supervisor should be aware of, and alert to, typical student errors

3. In connection with the supervisor's monitoring of patient responses (VIII, D, 2, d), special attention should be paid to the student's scoring of discrimination errors on a regular basis in the student's presence. This is necessary to determine if the student and supervisor are in agreement on the correctness of the patient's responses, particularly for monosyllabic word discrimination. It can be surprising to discover how often two people reach opposite conclusions. If the student seems to have a significant problem in this area, regular team monitoring/scoring is indicated

IX. Hearing aid selection

A. Pre-testing discussion with student

1. If patient has been seen in the clinic previously, particu-

larly for currently applicable audiometric testing, there is much to discuss, for example:

   a. Patient's background: history and communicative problems, and how they might serve as a guide in the hearing aid selection process

   b. What additional history information needs to be obtained

   c. Earphone test findings and their implications for hearing aid use

   d. Previous hearing aid use by patient: success in wearing amplification, type of aid, number of years worn, and the like

2. If patient has not been seen previously, decisions must be made regarding information provided by the otologic report, and then regarding what kinds of additional information should be obtained in detail: what to stress (communicative), what not to stress (medical)

3. After earphone testing is completed and/or supplemental history taken, discuss with student what will be done, for example:

   a. Approach to be used in unaided sound field testing

   b. Type(s) of amplification to be considered, and contributing factors

   c. Tests and test materials to be used

4. Depending on the case to be seen and time available, hearing aid specifications can be reviewed together with specific instruments being considered, before the patient is tested

All pre-testing discussion should be initiated and structured by supervisor for each case until he feels the student has internalized these steps and is able to proceed accordingly. The student's capabilities in this thinking process can be determined by asking him questions about his plans, with the eventual goal being completely independent deductions on the part of the student

B. Selection procedure

1. Demonstrate and discuss with student each step in the hearing aid selection process as he is exposed to it for the first time. (This is not to say that many, many repetitions will not be necessary.) Examples:

a. Choice of aid and settings, looking at specifications, considering unaided results
b. Choice of earmold: size, type; choice of tubing
c. Inserting earmold in patient's ear, putting aid on patient, coping with feedback problems
d. Setting, and necessary adjusting, of volume control
e. Informal evaluation of aided performance through talking with patient, asking him appropriate questions about his listening experiences
f. Knowing when to make a change in settings, mold, aid, or aided ear
g. Setting up test equipment:
    1. Choosing loudspeaker(s)
    2. Knowing when to omit, abbreviate, or include certain tests
h. Interpreting patient's subjective reactions to aids, and incorporating them meaningfully into the total picture
i. Considering nonaudiologic factors in selection and recommendation
j. Fielding patient's questions
k. Interpreting test findings: knowing when to stop testing; knowing what to recommend

Given the complexity of hearing aid selection and the variety of cases seen from week to week, the supervisor needs to observe the student very closely on all of these competencies. Even though the student may be able to perform a task relatively independently one week, he may not be able to do so the following week simply because the two cases are different. Thus, although it is important for the supervisor to see how well a student can modify and adapt his thinking and procedures from case to case, the supervisor must assist him in that very process by pointing out the similarities and differences among cases. This thinking process must be reinforced weekly

2. As in other areas, gradually fade away from the scene, leaving the student to work independently on the easiest tasks; that is, the ones with which he has had the most experience, such as the speech audiometry involved in testing of hearing aid performance

3. Continue to monitor all testing throughout the evaluation, however, so that problems can be detected and
solved immediately, because there is seldom enough time
to allow the luxury of retesting during a hearing aid selection procedure

4. Frequent spot checks are critical: inspect aids student has
put on patient to see if earmold is seated correctly, tubing
is not twisted, aid is not dangling, volume control is set
where the student thinks he has set it

   a. To accept test results in hearing aid selection without
   these spot checks is risky. However, the student
   should be made to understand that his work is being
   inspected not because the supervisor mistrusts him,
   but because of the great multitude of elusive variables in hearing aid work, and because seemingly
   small miscalculations can significantly alter the outcome of the selection procedure

   b. Spot checks should also be accompanied by explanation. That is to say, all the while the supervisor is
   checking, he should be telling and showing the
   student what he is looking for. This should prepare
   the student to do his own trouble-shooting in hearing
   aid work; at a later time the supervisor can ask the
   student to check certain items himself

5. Except in cases of straightforward hearing aid fittings,
maintain rather close surveillance of *all* students' hearing
aid selection work. Only through participatory involvement can the supervisor hope to achieve the goal of
teaching the student as much as possible within the time
allotted for this purpose. This is the point at which a relatively advanced student's step toward complete independence must be deferred, for several reasons:

   a. Because clinical hearing aid selection procedures are
   far from being totally objective, decisions are often
   based on experiential judgment; the supervisor has
   experience to rely on, the student does not. This
   should be carefully explained to the student who is
   anxious about his status of independence. To coun-
   terbalance this further, the student needs to be
   encouraged to contribute his own ideas as much as
   possible. If, and when, the student offers timely sug-

gestions or calls the supervisor's attention to any oversights, the student should be praised

b. Another reason for withholding complete student independence in hearing aid selection procedures is the student's lack of familiarity with:
   1. Community resources for referral and inquiry
   2. Local hearing aid dealers: their prices and policies
   3. Complete hearing aid stock in the clinical inventory

c. Finally, the patient must be able to identify with the person who will be in ultimate control of followup management, and that is the supervisor. Specifically, the patient must be aware of the fact that the supervisor took some part in the evaluation and has a good understanding of his problem, the test findings, and the recommendations

6. Serve as a model for the student in those activities that can, and should, be taught primarily in this manner, as:

   a. Recording information on the hearing aid worksheet and using it intelligently in comparing subjective and objective data. There usually is not sufficient time or need to discuss such accessory information in detail

   b. Talking to the patient throughout the evaluation: answering his questions knowledgeably, deciding when to say, "we will talk about that more, later on." (However, if a patient asks the student a question for which the student obviously has no answer or an inadequate answer, the supervisor should either interject a reply or subtly give the student the information he needs to relay to the patient. This is not a time to lose the patient's confidence in his clinicians. Regardless, all students need to be prepared for such occurrences in the event that the supervisor is absent from the test room when a question is asked. They should be advised to be honest with the patient, saying that they do not know the answer but will find out what it is; this is clearly preferable to feigning an answer which may later have to be retracted)

The supervisor has every right to expect the student to learn from these, and other, teaching models without having to make a point of explaining them in detail. But he also has the right to expect the student to ask questions during those moments when the student misunderstands something the supervisor has not taken the time to discuss. These expectations, of course, should have been clarified for the student during the orientation session as stated in I, B, 2. Finally, the supervisor has the right to expect the student to take notes when necessary

C.   Post-selection discussion, post-evaluation discussion
1.   Each case should be summarized in discussion with the student after completion of the test session. Unfortunately, there is not always enough time to do justice to this important review. Thus, the supervisor may not really know how well the student has integrated all of the factors in each case until the student's written account of the evaluation is submitted in the audiologic resumé. Nonetheless, when there is ample time, this dialogue should include:
     a.   Discussion of test findings and their implications
     b.   Discussion of the decision making that took place throughout the evaluation; that is, what steps were taken and why?
     c.   Discussion of the patient and his reactions to the evaluation, and how they affected the clinical decision-making process
     d.   Discussion of possible alternative actions; that is, what could have been done differently?
     This entire post-evaluation discussion should be structured to challenge the student's thinking, evaluate his progress since the previous week, and uncover his understanding weaknesses and strengths. It is an opportunity for both the supervisor and the student to reflect on their joint clinical efforts and perhaps find new meaning in the events that unfolded
2.   Case review should occur not only after evaluations involving audiologic management and followup, as in hearing aid selection, recheck, and orientation sessions, but after all audiologic testing whenever possible. This is often the supervisor's greatest opportunity for capitalizing on the wide variety of teaching points in each case.

A small sample of the range of topics which might be covered:

    a.   Typical/atypical symptomatologies

    b.   Interrelationships of symptoms reported by patients

    c.   Interrelationships of communicative problems reported by patients

    d.   Implications of intertest agreement/disagreement

    e.   Typical/atypical patient reactions to hearing aid use and their correlation with factors such as age, life style, degree and duration of hearing loss

  3. Keep student informed of post-evaluation management, and followup on recommendations by patients he has seen clinically

X. Counseling

  A. Patient counseling is the one area in which the supervisor needs to demonstrate by doing many, many times before the student assumes such responsibility. There are several reasons:

    1. The student needs to be exposed to the supervisor's adaptation of explanations to a wide variety of patients

    2. He needs to hear the supervisor answer patients' questions, structure counseling, and talk to patients' family members before he can be expected to do this himself

    3. He needs to have tested a number of patients before he can be expected to know how test results fit together and culminate in certain recommendations

    4. He needs to see and hear how the supervisor relates to patients and how the supervisor communicates with them

  B. Once the supervisor feels that the student has had enough exposure to counseling, the student can be brought into the act gradually, for example:

    1. The student can initially be asked to explain only the audiometric test results, while the supervisor does the remainder of the counseling

    2. During the next counseling opportunity, the student's participation can be expanded to include explanation of hearing aid test findings, while the supervisor discusses recommendations with the patient

    3. The final step in this gradual introduction would involve full student participation in the counseling process, but with the understanding that the supervisor may intervene

to answer questions that the student cannot handle, or to summarize at the end of the counseling session as the supervisor deems necessary

C. The alternative to a gradual immersion into the counseling process is full participation by the student on his first attempt. Such an approach works reasonably well with some students, especially those who have had brief counseling experiences in previous clinical assignments with other supervisors. For them, of course, the experience is not totally new, even though they are counseling under the direction of a new supervisor. Even so, these students should observe the counseling techniques of the current supervisor several times before beginning their own participation, because counseling varies among clinicians, and because the student should be given ample opportunity to observe his new model in action

D. Although the ideal sequence of counseling instruction might seem to be full student participation in the counseling of *every* patient after he has accomplished it completely by himself one time, my experience in this matter has proven otherwise

1. Because a student has not yet had exposure to every *type* of case, he has observed a limited number of counseling approaches. Therefore, the supervisor needs to assess each individual case in light of the student's counseling experience before a decision is reached as to who will do the counseling. If the supervisor determines that it would be more instructive for him to do the counseling than it would be for the student to do it, the reason behind this decision should be explained to the student before the counseling is begun

2. In some instances, the student may elect to forego participation in the counseling process because he feels he is not ready for it. When obviously difficult-to-counsel patients are under consideration, the supervisor might give the student a choice: full participation; team approach with supervisor (as detailed in X, B); or no active participation (that is, observation of the supervisor as model). Rarely have I disagreed with the student's decision regarding his readiness. (This is a clue to his self-evaluation capacity.) On those occasions of disagreement:

a. If the student feels he is capable of assuming the counseling responsibility independently, and the supervisor does not share his confidence, the supervisor may try to dissuade him. This course of action depends on many factors, such as student personality, type of patient, and time constraints. A frequently workable compromise: tell the student that he may begin the counseling, and that he will be given assistance if, and when, such is deemed necessary by the supervisor

b. If, on the other hand, the student does not feel he can handle the counseling of a particular patient but the supervisor thinks he can, he should be gently coaxed into trying, with the assurance that he will be given help if necessary. Some students undoubtedly need this "pushing" from the supervisor or they will not move forward in their clinical achievements; and, in fact, they are often pleasantly surprised to discover that they can do something they thought they were incapable of doing. Such a boost in self-confidence, along with supportive encouragement from the supervisor, is critically important to the student's growth

3. Whether the supervisor or the student conducts patient counseling, the supervisor should help the student to understand that he has much to gain from either experience. Indeed, it is difficult to determine which is the better learning experience in an area such as counseling. Although "learning by doing" is commonly thought to be more effective, this does not necessarily hold true in counseling; for example:

a. Will a student learn more by struggling through a counseling session with a patient quite unlike any he has ever counseled, or observed being counseled, or will he learn more through observation of the supervisor's counseling that patient? If the student serves as counselor in such a case, all the while making great errors of judgment, who will benefit? Certainly not the patient. And the student may not be aware of his errors until the supervisor later points them out. On the other hand, there is a great deal to be said for the viewpoint: "How will I know whether or not I can do it unless I am given the opportunity to try?"

b.   Needless to say, the decision of whether or not to counsel is sometimes a difficult one for the supervisor and student to reach. But, if at all possible, they should make this decision together, with mutual understanding of the other's feelings on the matter

c.   A final comment on this issue needs to be made here: a big factor in a supervisor's occasional reluctance to allow the student full counseling responsibility is the supervisor's unwillingness to have his patient receive counseling that he believes to be of lesser quality than his own. This is understandable, but not acceptable: a supervisor who has committed himself to teaching must be willing to make this compromise, as well as many others

E.   All patient counseling sessions, whether carried out by the supervisor, the student, or both parties, should be preceded by some type of preparatory discussion of what the counseling will involve:

1.   This should include discussion of what will be emphasized in the counseling session, and what will be omitted or handled cursorily. That is to say, what approach will be used with a particular patient and for what reasons?

2.   If the student is going to conduct the counseling, he should be encouraged to take some notes with him into the session if he thinks he might forget certain points to be covered with the patient. For some students, the mere availability of such an aid fosters a feeling of security

3.   Prestructure the counseling session for the student until he is able to do this by himself. This can be done only in somewhat general terms, of course, because there is no way of knowing in advance precisely what questions the patient will ask or how he will respond to the counseling. The supervisor may be able to anticipate some interactions, however, in the light of his foreknowledge about the patient's behavior during the earlier parts of the audiologic evaluation. Thus, he can prepare the student with some probabilities, for example:

a.   "If the patient says ＿＿, what will you say?" He can give the student some sample answers

      b. "Explain the hearing aid testing in this way," giving him the words to say almost verbatim

F. During the student's counseling, the supervisor should listen closely from an adjacent room. He also needs to observe from time to time as the student is interacting with the patient, although this should be done with some discretion so the student does not become inhibited[3]

  1. Through observation, the supervisor can see:

    a. If the student is facing the patient, enunciating clearly for lipreading purposes

    b. How the student addresses family members

    c. Student's facial expressions

    d. How student handles unexpected hearing aid problems (for example, feedback)

    e. How student points to audiogram features or other pictorial/written material when illustrating a point

  2. Through attentive listening, the supervisor can quickly pinpoint student difficulties. Depending on their gravity, the supervisor should feel free to intervene. Although it may appear to be disruptive (the student, of course, should have been forewarned of this possible occurrence), it is sometimes necessary and often preferable to the supervisor's addition of counseling points out of context after the student has finished his discussion with the patient. This is a difficult supervisory decision, and a useful rule of thumb is: intervene if the addition/correction of information is necessary at that point in order to ensure that the remainder of the counseling session will be meaningful. To be sure, the supervisor must be self-restraining, as the desire to intervene unnecessarily and take control of the situation is often difficult to repress

G. All counseling sessions should be followed by a post-mortem discussion between supervisor and student. This should be included in the total post-evaluation discussion as described in IX, C. The following points need to be covered:

  1. The patient's reaction to the counseling

  2. What was good about the counseling and what could have been better

  3. How the student felt about his own counseling, or how the supervisor felt about his own counseling. The supervisor should point out to the student that he does not

---

[3] Observation areas with one-way glass can do much to alleviate this problem.

always experience a feeling of complete satisfaction with his own patient counseling, because perfection is virtually unattainable in this area, hence the need for perpetual self-evaluation

XI. Resumé and Report Writing[4]

    A. Instruction on audiologic resumé[5] and report writing should be handled by the supervisor during the post-mortem discussion of each case

        1. An explanation of the purpose of resumés (that is, how they are utilized by an on-the-job audiologist) should be given to beginning clinical students and, if necessary, reviewed for nonbeginners. This explanation can be supported by illustrative examples of how resumé entries are instrumental in ongoing patient management

        2. The beginner can be given a sample resumé to use as a guideline when he attempts to write his first one for each type of assignment

        3. The student should be told what format is used for typing resumés and reports, how they will be edited by the supervisor and then returned to the student

        4. Prestructuring of each resumé and report is necessary until the supervisor determines that the student no longer needs this preparation. This should include discussion matters such as:

            a. What points need to be brought out in the resumé for a particular patient

            b. Who will be receiving the report and what kind of information needs to be conveyed to the intended recipient. The supervisor must stress the importance of adapting one's writing of reports to suit the varying levels of sophistication and informational needs of the readers

            c. After such detailed instruction has taken place for several weeks, the supervisor can be more general in this preparatory discussion so that the student has to begin making his own decisions regarding the structure and style of a report as well as specific statements within it

---

[4] All our students in clinical practicum assignments are required to author any written work associated with their cases.

[5] Audiological resumé is our term for the written chronological account of history, test findings, and management included in the records of all patients whose evaluations generate sufficient information to warrant such a summary.

d. The ultimate supervisory goal is to provide no prestructuring assistance for the student. As with counseling and other highly professional skills, however, perfection is really never achieved. Thus, there is nearly always a need for some kind of preliminary discussion. Regardless of this continuing need, the supervisor should make every attempt to shift the decision making responsibility to the student as they collaborate on writing strategies

e. Although the provision of sample reports for students is oftentimes instructive, particularly when a specific writing style or format is required, the use of such aids can quickly stifle creative writing bents. Once a student has been taught the fundamentals of clinical report writing and is armed with the supervisor's suggestions for approaching the writing of an assigned report, the student will learn a great deal more if he is faced with a blank piece of paper than he will with a sample report at his side. The latter discourages independent thinking and the choice of one's own words, both necessary ingredients in the development of writing proficiency. Moreover, a recognized key to good writing is diligent, daily practice (Pannbacker, 1975). The indiscriminate use of report guides and samples not only precludes originality in writing but perpetuates some of the well-known shortcomings in clinical reports: pat phrases, stilted wording, and unnecessary use of jargon

f. The student should be encouraged to read his reports aloud after writing them, to determine if they flow smoothly, are well organized, and make good sense. Such an exercise is often revealing and can help the student to detect his own writing weaknesses[6]

---

[6] For further information on report writing, the reader is referred to the recently published Report Writing in the Field of Communication Disorders by Kenneth J. Knepflar (1976). This handbook, sponsored by the National Student Speech and Hearing Association, should be examined by every supervisor and his student clinicians; the supervisor would also be well advised to study some of the references in its bibliography to enhance his own writing skills. As Pannbacker (1975) has noted, clinical supervisors are almost solely responsible for the teaching of report writing in our field.

B. Editing of resumés and reports
1. The actual editing of student-prepared resumés and reports constitutes one of the supervisor's most time-consuming and painstaking jobs
2. The supervisor must make compromises in editing. That is to say, the final product may not be written in exactly the same way it would have been had the entire responsibility of authorship belonged exclusively to the supervisor. Nonetheless, even if the wording is not his own, the ideas contained in any student-prepared, supervisor-edited report obviously should reflect the supervisor's thinking; it is he who signs the report and he who must bear the ultimate responsibility for its contents
3. All editing should include explanations and comments for the student in the margins, unless the supervisor is certain he will have the opportunity to discuss his editing in detail with the student
4. The editing supervisor should be meticulous in his correction of punctuation, spelling and grammatical errors. It is unfortunate that some students at the graduate school level have not yet mastered these basic skills, but such is the case. The clinical supervisor is typically the last person who has the opportunity to teach some of these rudiments to a student before the student enters the professional world
5. In general, the supervisor can be less exacting in editing of resumés than he can afford to be with report editing. The reason is quite obvious: reports are sent outside the clinic for public consumption, whereas resumés are kept in patients' clinical files for use by staff members. Although this relaxing of editorial duties lessens the supervisor's work load somewhat, it does not diminish his responsibility to the student. For example, if certain portions of the resumé are left unedited with the knowledge that they could have been stated better, the supervisor should call this to the student's attention with an accompanying explanation of how the wording might have been improved

C. Discussion of edited written work
1. The supervisor should make every attempt to have a student's edited written work returned to the student within two weeks after the patient's appointment, or at

the end of one week if possible. In order to accomplish this, the student's deadline for turning in completed work needs to be set for no more than a few days after the appointment to allow for editing and typing. There are sound reasons for imposing such time restrictions:

    a.   All reports should be sent to referring sources and other interested parties as soon as possible

    b.   Both the student and the supervisor should work on reports and resumés while the evaluation is easily recalled, and discuss the edited written work with the patient still firmly in mind

    c.   It is to the supervisor's advantage to bring the student's errors to his attention as soon as possible

    d.   It is to the student's advantage to know how he is faring in his written work, and then to concentrate on improving his skills as soon as possible

2.   The supervisor should make an attempt to discuss each piece of returned written work with the student

    a.   This can be accomplished at any time, before or after a clinic session, or during a conference between supervisor and student. However, for instruction purposes, the best time is during the preparatory prestructuring discussion for writing up a current case, because the student will derive optimum learning from this combination

    b.   The supervisor should encourage student questions during such discussion. Once certain problems have been identified, the supervisor can offer appropriate suggestions, including outside reading assignments on the topic of writing

D.   Exceptions to the rule

1.   For a beginning clinical student involved in a basic audiometric testing assignment, it is not reasonable to assign the writing of clinical reports until that student has demonstrated he is ready for this task. The supervisor can judge the student's readiness by taking into consideration the number and quality of resumés he has produced and his overall understanding of clinical work. This gradual introduction to report writing, in accordance with the skill/competency scales, is often more conducive to learning, and less confusing, for the student

2.   If the supervisor elects not to have the student write a

given report, but instead does it himself, he should provide the student with a copy of the work, and then discuss it with the student in detail

XII. Evaluation

A. As stated in Chapter 3, evaluation of the student's clinical performance is an ongoing process, the result of supervisory observation and analysis. The following sections contain representative questions which arise from observation and analysis, and then culminate in evaluation. These are merely examples of the kinds of questions a supervisor must answer in his own mind, and they do not cover all areas of evaluation

1. Review of medical records and other patient information

   a. Does student understand terminology?

   b. Is student capable of seeing relationships among different informational factors?

   c. Can student reach logical conclusions on the basis of available information?

   d. Can student determine which information is useful to him and which is not?

2. Patient interview

   a. Does student phrase questions so that the patient understands what he is asking? Can he adapt terminology to the patient's level of understanding?

   b. Is student able to communicate effectively with patients having severe hearing losses?

   c. Does student relate warmly and compassionately to patients?

   d. Is student flexible in his questioning, showing an ability to follow the patient's responses, or is he rigid and tied to the order of questions on his history form? Can student pursue supplementary questioning in those areas where necessary, or is his repertoire limited to the questions printed on his history form? Is the student fluent in his questioning?

   e. How effectively does the student include family members in his interview of the patient?

   f. How well does the student record information?

      1. Is information recorded in the appropriate blanks?

2. Does information make sense when read, or is it sketchy, confusing, and/or meaningless?
3. Is handwriting legible?
4. Does student translate patient's replies into professional terminology when recording, or is he tied to the patient's wording? Does student know when it is important to record patient's answers verbatim and when it is not?

g. Can the student pace himself in history-taking and accomplish the task within a reasonable period of time?
h. Can he tactfully lead a rambling, verbose patient back to the topic of discussion?

3. Pure tone audiometry
   a. Does student know how to employ Hughson-Westlake method (Carhart and Jerger, 1959), or whatever method the supervisor adopts, and when to deviate from it if indicated?
   b. Is student capable of establishing accurate thresholds?
   c. Does he make logical decisions in threshold pursuit when patient's responses are somewhat inconsistent and/or the final threshold is in question?
   d. Does he know what to do when responses are erratic?
   e. Can he work quickly without compromising accuracy?
   f. Can he judge test reliability?

4. Masking
   a. Does he know when to mask?
   b. Does he know how to employ the Hood technique (1960), or whatever technique the supervisor adopts, and when to deviate from it if indicated?
   c. Does he recognize overmasking problems and know how to cope with them?
   d. Does he understand the use of masking in suprathreshold testing?

5. Speech audiometry
   a. Does student familiarize patient with test words correctly, and know when and how to deviate from the conventional procedure if indicated?

      b. Does student know how to use Tillman-Olsen method (1972), or whatever method the supervisor adopts, and when to deviate from it if indicated?

      c. Does student know when the use of monitored live voice is indicated?

      d. Can he carry out monitored live voice testing well?

      e. Does student know when to modify test procedures, for example, SAT instead of SRT, use of selected spondees, elimination of carrier phrase, use of special speech materials, use of half lists?

      f. Can student make logical decisions in selecting presentation levels for discrimination testing?

6. Hearing aid selection

      a. Is student able to determine what types of amplification are appropriate for each case?

      b. Does student consider the appropriate factors in selecting specific instruments?

      c. Can he manipulate hearing aid controls, batteries, earmolds?

      d. Does he know what questions to ask patients in ascertaining their subjective reactions to hearing aids?

      e. Does he know what factors indicate the need for a change in his course of action?

      f. Does he make logical decisions in choosing tests for hearing aid evaluation?

      g. Does he reach the appropriate conclusions in making hearing aid recommendations?

7. Counseling

      a. Is student able to assess the patient's needs, then make appropriate decisions on the approach he will use in counseling?

      b. How well does student relate to patient, family members? Is he "professional?"

      c. Is student fluent in his counseling? Natural? Relaxed? Convincing?

      d. Are his explanations clear? Sufficient in depth and scope?

      e. Is his counseling session well structured? Is there smooth transition from topic to topic?

      f. Can student adapt his terminology and structure to meet the patient's needs while he is counseling; that is, how well does student "read" the patient's reactions and respond accordingly?

   g. How well can student field patient's questions?

8. Resumé and report writing

   a. Do student's resumés reflect an integrated understanding of the patient's problems, test results and clinical decisions made during the evaluation? Check for:

     1. Accurate statement of test findings

     2. Logical conclusions

     3. Observations of patient behavior

   b. Are resumés and reports well written? Check for:

     1. Use of professional terminology, vocabulary level

     2. Creativity, variety in writing style

     3. Sentence construction

     4. Clarity of ideas

     5. Continuity (chronological ordering of events), cohesiveness

     6. Conciseness

     7. Appropriateness of choice of topics to be included or excluded, explained in detail or mentioned only briefly

     8. Spelling, grammar, punctuation

   c. Does student learn from corrected errors on previous written work or does he repeat them?

   d. Is work handed in on time?

   e. Is work neat?

9. General

   a. How easily, accurately can student operate test equipment?

   b. Are test instructions clear?

   c. Can student interpret test results, and then make appropriate clinical decisions on the basis of this determination?

   d. Does student know when to make recommendations other than hearing aid use? Does he know when to make referrals to other services?

   e. How does student relate to supervisor and supervision? Does student accept criticism?

   f. Does student have ample initiative, or does he have to be told everything to do?

   g. What is student's attitude toward clinical work?

     h.   Does student improve in his clinical performance from week to week, quarter to quarter?

     i.   Does student ask pertinent questions of supervisor?

     j.   How accurately and thoroughly does student fill out forms?

B.   Because the supervisor has so many competencies to evaluate for each student and because it is not possible to complete an evaluation form at the conclusion of each week's test session, it is helpful to keep some type of weekly diary or record of each student's progress. This can be accomplished rather easily by devising a grid, with competencies heading the vertical columns and dates of clinical practicum sessions listed down the left-hand side. The supervisor can then record brief notes in the appropriate spaces, using some sort of ranking system or whatever is most meaningful. Unless this kind of record-keeping is done, it is virtually impossible to remember accurately how a student performs in each area from week to week. And if the supervisor has difficulty recalling at the end of the quarter exactly what kinds of improvements the student has attained in each area, the final written evaluation will consequently be less than fair or accurate

C.   Evaluation is just as important for the student's sake as it is for the supervisor's sake; therefore, the supervisor must keep him informed as to his progress. Because there is rarely time to have weekly conferences and it is probably not even reasonable to have detailed weekly evaluation discussion, the supervisor can accomplish this in an informal, unstructured manner. Indeed, the student is being informed of his progress in each area during the many discussions the supervisor has with him before, during, and after a test session. For example:

     1.   Observation of the student's testing enables the supervisor to give him suggestions, point out his errors and how to correct them, or praise him for a job well done. This constitutes evaluation, in that the student is being told in various ways just how he measures up to the supervisor's expectations

     2.   Weekly review of written work with the student includes explanation of his strengths and weaknesses. This also constitutes up-to-date evaluation of the student's progress

A comment should be made here about the student's concept

of ongoing evaluation and feedback. A significant number of the students in our program have over the years suggested that they were not being kept informed of their progress on a weekly basis. My own personal view of their feelings on this matter is that they have a misconception of what weekly evaluation and feedback should be. Their base of reference is coursework where each evaluation yields a grade and the students know their exact status at any given time following such evaluations. Clinical evaluations, on the other hand, are too complex for weekly precision of this sort and, furthermore, weekly grading would be meaningless. In view of this example of an apparent discrepancy between students' and supervisors' conceptions of what constitutes ongoing evaluation and feedback, it is important that the supervisor explain his evaluation procedure to students

D. In addition to the weekly informal evaluation events, the supervisor should have an evaluation conference with the student at midterm time. Although this does not have to include a written evaluation, it should be a summary review with the student of:
   1. His progress since the beginning of the quarter
   2. Whether or not his progress is satisfactory to the supervisor
   3. His areas of strength and weakness
   4. How the student feels about his clinical performance, the clinical assignment in general, and whether or not he would like the supervisor to alter the teaching approach to help him learn better

   If a student is having special problems in his clinical work, of course, the supervisor should not limit the number of evaluation conferences to the midterm and final meetings, but should have as many such discussions as he and the student deem necessary

E. The final conference includes review and discussion of the written evaluation[7] by supervisor and student. This is

---

[7] See Appendix I for a sample of the student clinician evaluation form currently used in our audiology program. The latest version in a series of changing forms over many years, it represents what we believe to be a successful compromise between previously used, and discarded, subjective and objective evaluation methods. (The first sections on professionalism were designed to mutually serve students in other clinical areas of our program.) In spite of its proven utility, the form continues to be evaluated periodically and is now undergoing further revision.

Students are familiarized with the details of this evaluation form in their clinical seminars.

probably best accomplished by:

1. Reading together with the student the rating and comments on each item in the evaluation

2. Explaining to the student the reasoning behind these remarks. The citing of specific examples of the student's work is helpful here if the supervisor's memory and notes are adequate

3. Encouraging the student to respond to each item; that is, finding out if he feels the supervisor's appraisal is similar to his self-evaluation. If the student disagrees with the rating, this should be discussed; and if there is a great discrepancy between the supervisor's and student's opinions on a certain item, the supervisor should add the student's remarks to the evaluation form for the record[8]

4. Encouraging the student to express his feelings on why he is performing poorly or well in each area. This can be followed by a discussion of ways in which he might strive to improve poor performance or capitalize on good performance. The supervisor should do less talking and more listening here, to maximize the student's opportunity for contributing his own ideas. Such open, balanced discussion is quite meaningful for both the supervisor and student:

   a. For the supervisor: it helps him to capsulize further the student's current status in clinical practicum, thereby enabling the supervisor to make more incisive comments during staffing and scheduling of the student for subsequent clinical assignments

   b. For the student: it allows him to engage in critical self-evaluation, an all-important thought process for every student clinician. (If the supervisor has been doing his job throughout the quarter, he will have already instilled in the student some ability to pursue self-analysis of clinical behavior.) This is the time for the student to reflect on where he is going, and if he still wants to go. This type of discussion

---

[8] After a student clinician evaluation has been discussed, and signed, by student and supervisor, it is forwarded to a coordinator who averages the clinical grade with other clinical grades earned by the student during the quarter, thereby culminating in a single grade for the clinical study registration. The evaluation form is then entered in the student's personal record on file with the audiology program. The student may have a personal copy of his evaluation on request.

can become very personal in nature, and the supervisor should handle it as such: he should be supportive but honest

5. Following the detailed review of individual items on the evaluation form, the supervisor should summarize for the student his strengths and weaknesses, then comment on their implications for his needs in future clinical assignments, whether these be in the university training program, in an externship setting, or in a job setting following graduation

6. Final discussion will center on the letter grade that the supervisor has given the student. The supervisor should explain what factors helped him to reach this decision. These should include:

   a. Self-comparison: how does the student's current performance compare to his previous performance, both at the beginning of this quarter, and in previous quarters under this supervisor's guidance? In short, how has he progressed?

   b. Peer comparison: how does his performance compare with that of his classmates who are at similar stages in the clinical training process? Is he lagging behind, on a par with them, or relatively advanced?

   c. Supervisory judgment: is the student performing at a level expected by the supervisor of someone with his given background of clinical and academic preparation? Were the goals stated at the beginning of the quarter reached?

   d. Method of grading: how does the supervisor derive a grade? That is, how are evaluative judgments translated into the assigned letter grade?

F. Some final comments need to be made here about the written evaluation itself:

1. The supervisor will have less difficulty in ranking the student on each item if his observations and notes throughout the clinical assignment have been thorough

2. Written comments on the form should be as detailed as possible so that they are useful to all who may read them:

   a. The student, who deserves to know in detail his clinical strengths and weaknesses

   b. The supervisor, for future reference. Indeed, he

might want to make copies of these evaluations for his individual future use

1. If he has the same student again in a future clinical assignment, he can make evaluative comparisons, thus enabling him to determine if the student has progressed, stayed at the same level, or regressed

2. He needs this information if he is called upon to write a letter of recommendation for a student

c. Other supervisors, who may have the student in future clinical assignments. They need to know the student's level of performance to help decide their supervisory approach

d. The student's academic adviser, who needs to have an accurate picture of the student's clinical work so that he can advise the student intelligently

3. Written comments should include positive remarks as well as negative remarks, with reasonable balance between the two if at all possible. Criticism should be constructive and worded carefully, although honesty should never be compromised

CHAPTER 5

THE TRAINING OF SUPERVISORS IN AUDIOLOGY

CONTENTS

The need for formal training of supervisors has been recognized by the majority of those individuals and groups who have addressed the topic of supervision in communicative disorders. As noted in the introductory chapter, such training has been initiated by some university training programs; one of these is the Department of Communicative Disorders at Northwestern University. Notwithstanding the existence of a workshop for supervisors of speech and language pathology programs, audiology personnel in the department developed a supervisor training component to serve the specific needs of audiologists. In its third year of operation, this project has evolved in three distinct modes: a course on audiology supervision for advanced graduate students in the clinical training program; inservice training for on-campus and off-campus supervisors; and supervision practicum for staff supervisors in training. This chapter is devoted to a report of our experiences in these endeavors.

AUDIOLOGY SUPERVISION COURSE FOR STUDENTS

Our course in audiology supervision for students has now completed its third round. The previously described weekly clinical seminar was chosen as the most likely entry point into the curriculum for an experimental course of this type. Thus, two hours per week for an entire school quarter (ten weeks in this instance) are spent in the classroom. In addition to these twenty hours of instruction and discussion, more time is required for outside projects assigned in connection with the course. The participating students have been those in their fifth or sixth quarter of clinical study registration, thereby giving us a class composition of second-year master's students (during the quarter immediately preceding their externship assignments and graduation) and doctoral students still

A condensed version of the material in this chapter was presented at the Annual Convention of the American Speech and Hearing Association, Chicago (1977).

enrolled in the clinical study sequence. The course was designed by me and, during its pilot year, taught with the assistance of another on-campus supervisor. Since that initial trial run, I have become the sole instructor.

The students have approached this course with a variety of anticipatory feelings. Some state that they aspire to eventual supervisory roles in their upcoming careers, and others express a hope that they will never be called upon to supervise. In spite of this dichotomy, all see the need for a course in the training of supervisors. This attitude is reinforced when they are reminded that supervisory responsibilities are encountered in many job settings outside the realm of a university training program; for example: sponsorship of a CFY trainee; off-campus supervision at the request of a university training facility; orientation of new staff members; training, or overseeing the work of, audiometric technicians, nurses, et al.; or carrying out the administrative duties of a clinical directorship. Even though the course is based on a university-oriented, clinical teaching concept, it was our hope that each student would derive some practical benefit from this experience.

The core material presented in the course is essentially equivalent to the contents of Chapters 1 through 4 herein, and therefore actually laid the groundwork for this book. The bibliography, also similar to the one presented here, was compiled after selecting primarily those readings which seemed to have some relevance to supervision in audiology. From the bibliography list, references are further culled and assigned to students for outside reading, abstraction, and class presentation. Class discussions thus have revolved around information from two sets of sources: experiential contributions regarding audiology supervision per se from the students and supervisor/instructor; and nonaudiology material on supervision from within and without the field of communicative disorders. Although some of the outside source material has proven to be of questionable relevance to the course's specific concerns, the combined sources offer a meaningful blend of thought-provoking and discussion-stimulating information. Class deliberation also has centered around primarily student-submitted "questions, problems, issues" that are requested the first day of class, and then openly discussed during the final class meetings. This material is divided into categories, such as interpersonal relationships, evaluation of supervisors, and evaluation of students, and then assigned to small groups for preclass analysis before they are required to lead class debate on the chosen topic areas. This activity has been especially productive, because it focuses on the individual concerns of all of the participants.

In keeping with the combined lecture/seminar format of this course, two additional class participation segments were introduced in its second year. These changes constituted part of, and were made possible by, the reorganization process deemed appropriate on the basis of interim course evaluation. The first course modification, a group exercise in the editing of a poorly written audiologic report, proved to be a useful supplement to the formal presentation on this area of supervisory responsibility. The second course modification, a session requiring class members to interact in predetermined student/supervisor roles, was equally contributory to the discussion of interpersonal relationships.

Projects assigned for out-of-class completion are directed toward more individual endeavors. In one of these, the students are asked to listen to audiotaped supervision sessions with an accompanying printed guide to the taped activities and with copies of related patient records. The four and one-half hours of taped material was prepared in various kinds of supervisory activities, including different types of clinical assignments, a broad sample of clinical competencies, and supervision of students at different levels in the practicum sequence. The associated guide, excerpts of which are shown in Appendix II, describes in detail the following types of information: clinical activity; physical setting/location of participants; patient code (for reference to patient records); clinical competency being taught; level of participating student; and step-by-step account, both method and rationale, of the audiotaped supervision process. In essence, then, this guide represents an applied, more specific version of the basic model of audiology supervision offered in Chapter 4. The students are encouraged to bring back to class any questions or comments that might occur to them as they contemplate the material. This plan works rather well, and the students seem particularly appreciative of having the opportunity to read about the taped sessions before actually listening to them, so that they can devote their full attention to the developing taped events. Furthermore, they can listen to the material (recorded on audiocassettes) in small groups of twos and threes, thereby enabling them to discuss matters more readily. And, as hoped, some of these observational experiences have prompted questions that come to the fore in class discussion.

The remaining two class projects involve the introduction of students to supervision practicum. In the first such assignment, each student is required to supervise the course instructor as that instructor plays the role of a beginning clinical student. Although the original plan was to use actual patients, the clinic schedule could not accommodate this added activity. Therefore, staff members were called on to play the parts of "patients." They have assumed their acting roles so convincingly (losses range from high-frequency unilaterals to conductive bilaterals; reported histories are replete with pathological symptoms) that the "student" (instructor) and "supervisors" (students) frequently have more realism than expected. Moreover, the use of staff members as "patients" affords much more flexibility, particularly in the manipulation of test/time factors, and the practicing supervisors can operate under less pressure than they would if real patients were involved. The objective of this project assignment is to give student supervisors an opportunity to go through the paces of supervising a naive clinical student, someone they need to instruct in the fundamentals of audiometric testing. Actual beginning clinical students are not used because this activity is undertaken after the middle of the school quarter, and because it is important that the student supervisors first be exposed to the audiotaped model and class discussion of supervisory methodology for basic competencies. Furthermore, participation as "student" allows the course instructor to evaluate the student supervisors' skills in the four areas that they are told will be examined: (1) knowledge of what to include in basic instruction for a beginning student; (2) clarity of explanation; (3) detection of student's errors; and (4) ability to handle student's questions.

The working premise is explained to each student supervisor in this manner: the supervision practicum session is designed to include preparation for, and the testing and counseling of, one "patient"; the "student" is to be approached as though having had one practicum session preceding the current one. Following the assigned supervision practicum session, evaluative comments, suggestions, and criticism are recorded by the course instructor in the four areas noted above and for each clinical activity. The grid used for this evaluation, shown with sample comments in Appendix III, is subsequently returned to each student in order to provide him with a permanent, detailed critique of his supervisory skills under the specified conditions. Some oral critical comments are also made during, and immediately after, the sessions. Most students have reacted quite favorably to this venture; a few report that the experience is somewhat intimidating and therefore precludes optimum learning. All are astonished by the time and energy demands and the overall complexity of the task.

The second supervision practicum assignment, scheduled to take place (insofar as possible) on a date some time after the activity just described, involves supervision of an actual student in the presence of an actual patient undergoing an actual audiologic evaluation. This is accomplished by assigning a student supervisor to work in an already supervised clinical activity that ordinarily is staffed by the course instructor and a first-year master's student. At the time of this special assignment, the regular supervisor participates only in an advisory capacity, thereby giving the student supervisor as much freedom as he can reasonably manage. He is checked primarily on patient management decisions, but otherwise left alone to supervise his student. As with the first supervision practicum assignment, the student supervisor's responsibilities are limited to the audiologic evaluation of one patient. In each instance, the first-year master's student is coached for his upcoming involvement with a student supervisor. Because of scheduling conflicts and the inflexibility of clinic schedules, some of these students are necessarily subjected to more than one student supervisor, but attempts are made to hold this to a minimum. Because the course instructor is involved in this student-supervised activity in a peripheral manner to reduce any potential inhibitory factor, the student supervisors are not evaluated directly. Instead, they are evaluated on the quality of their written reports of this supervisory experience. Appendix IV shows the sample outline that is provided to guide them in the report preparation. As indicated, the student supervisors are required not only to give a detailed account of their first real supervisory endeavor, but also to develop a multifaceted analysis of its dynamics.

The resultant papers have been fascinating. The students in the supervision course have succeeded in pulling together many of the aspects of audiology supervision covered in class as they see them materialize in their supervision practicum assignments. They have offered observations of their supervisory experiences that are extraordinarily insightful for novices. And, paralleling reactions to the supervision practicum role-playing activity, this experience evokes an almost unanimous comment about the complexity of supervision, with many students remarking that it proved to be much more difficult than anticipated. For a number of students, the experience helps to crystallize thinking on aspirations to supervise eventually. All in all, this part of the supervision practicum project represents a fitting culmination to the course. As time permits, a class discussion is held to give the student supervisors an opportunity to exchange their ideas on this supervision practicum experience.

There are no written examinations in the course. Rather, the final grade is based on: the abstraction of assigned readings (handed in by each student, then graded and photocopied for class distribution) and the corresponding oral presentation; the previously described supervisory competencies in the practicum role-playing assignment; and the report on supervision practicum with a student of lesser experience. An evaluation sheet with explanatory comments is provided for each student. The mean grade derived from these three components is then averaged with each student's other clinical (practicum) grades for the school quarter, resulting in a single overall grade for the clinical study registration.

Course evaluations are distributed at the final class meeting with a request that they be completed at a later time, after the students have been notified of their grades. Although the evaluation form has already undergone considerable revision since its first year of use, attempts are still being made to probe in some detail those areas considered germane to this experimental teaching venture. Among these are: the contribution of such a course to the curriculum in an audiology clinical training program; course content; class discussion; bibliography; assigned readings; taped supervision sessions; supervision practicum assignments; evaluation/grading system; and the overall impact of the course.

Following the pilot year, responses to individual items varied greatly, ranging from total acceptance to guarded rejection of certain aspects of the course. More importantly, all included feasible suggestions for modification and, as alluded to earlier, a number of changes were made in the course for its second run. The more recent evaluations reflect apparent improvement, as essentially all facets of the course are now being well received. Without exception, each year's respondents have been in agreement on the single most important matter: they feel that the course is a valuable addition to the audiology training program. We are heartened by this collective response and will proceed accordingly. The course will continue to be offered, with further experimental changes when deemed appropriate.

This experience has strongly reinforced our support of those Schubert minimal requirements for supervisors that call for supervision practicum and academic course work in supervision (1974).

INSERVICE TRAINING FOR ON-CAMPUS
AND OFF-CAMPUS SUPERVISORS

Although we have long recognized a need for inservice training, or continuing education, in audiology supervision for our staff supervisory personnel at Northwestern University, little concerted effort was made in this direction until quite recently. Past endeavors were limited to infrequent discussions of clinical technique; for example, methods of determining speech reception thresholds, uniformity in the use of audiometric symbols, and the clinical application of masking. Occasionally, time was devoted to in-depth deliberation of a particular student "problem" during quarterly student scheduling meetings. And, on two occasions, a staff psychologist explored the dynamics of interpersonal relationships as they pertain to clinical supervision. Notwithstanding the importance of these efforts to improve supervision, they seemed to occur only when special needs arose or when someone suggested that group examination of a particular area might be mutually beneficial. In other words, the approach to improving supervision from within the training program's ranks was both random and inadequate.

Fortunately, several forces converged during the past few years that compelled a look at this issue in a different light. As indicated in the description of the clinical practicum system in Chapter 4, the program began using more off-campus practicum sites than it has in the past. This situation naturally involved new supervisors, supervisors who had never supervised before, supervisors in settings that differed markedly from university clinics, supervisors who were totally unfamiliar with Northwestern's training program. In addition, new supervisors were added to the on-campus staff. And finally, experiences in the supervision course for students left no room for doubt; frank class discussions of supervision problems, as viewed by the students, uncovered a clear need for inservice training. Even though there had been a vehicle for student evaluation of supervisors for some time,[1] it was never as revealing as the unprecedented oral and written comments that emanated from the supervision course.

With ample incentive, then, we proceeded with plans for initiating a systematic approach to inservice training and/or ongoing education of our on-campus and off-campus audiology supervisors. The first step was undertaken at a regular practicum scheduling meeting that followed the initial course on supervision for students. Nearly all of the 15 program supervisors were present. Following an overview of the just-completed course and a brief presentation on the increasing interest in supervisor training in communicative disorders, the group was polled to find out who might be interested in pursuing such a venture. Everyone was receptive to the proposal, particularly the off-campus supervisors. Accordingly, arrangements were made to send each supervisor a packet of pertinent materials, all of which had been produced for, or resulted from, the supervision course for the students. In addition, the audiocassettes and associated patient information that had been used in the students' course were sent to the supervisors. As explained beforehand to all the participants, the hope was that this material would stimulate thinking

---

[1] The form currently in use for student evaluation of audiology supervisors, supervision, and practicum assignments is displayed in Appendix V. Like its counterpart in Appendix I, this form was recently revised to fulfill a common need by different clinical areas in our program (professionalism sections on pages 123 and 124). It was designed also to match in format the evaluation used by supervisors to appraise students.

about supervision, promote self-analysis of supervisory work, and most importantly, generate questions that could later be submitted for group consideration and discussion.

After a quarter had passed, the supervisors began submitting their own questions and concerns about supervision. The first supervision seminar was then scheduled. During the interim, the supervisors' questions were grouped into categories, pre-assigned for analysis and discussion prior to the seminar (as had been done with this activity in the students' course), and then returned as a completed set of discussion topics to the participants. Although there was some duplication among the questions submitted, they easily covered the range of possible concerns in audiology supervision. The questions were excellent, probing in nature, and very few could be answered conclusively. Thus, they provided the group with discussion material ideally suited for debate. And, if any skepticism about the need for guidance in supervision still remained, these expressed concerns of both experienced and inexperienced supervisors confirmed the wisdom of inservice training plans. The final draft of 75 distinct questions/concerns, prepared by ten different supervisors, resulted in the following breakdown: methodology; availability of supervisory time; evaluation of students and of supervisors; interpersonal relationships; building student independence; training of supervisors; concerns about off-campus supervision; and a miscellaneous grouping for unclas.ifiable items.

Despite realization of the monumental task ahead, the seminar proceedings were conducted unhurriedly and with deliberation; it mattered not how much ground was covered, but rather how substantive the discussion would be. With this as a guidepost, a four-hour discourse on the enigma of audiology supervision was initiated. The conversation was fairly uninhibited and free-flowing, and moved from one topic area to another quite naturally. And, not surprisingly, only nine of the 75 stated items were addressed within the allotted time. However, the efforts were productive, and the time well spent. Each participant contributed to the exchange of ideas, and each benefited from this exchange. The session was more therapeutic than informative, more inspiring than instructive, but ·it was a start. The dialogue had begun. Everyone agreed that this joint exploration of issues in audiology supervision should be continued.

Since that auspicious beginning, the seminars have been held at quarterly intervals, even more often when participants have requested such. The interest level remains high. Although the group has digressed from the original list of concerns, this in itself has been productive. Specifically, at the suggestion of one of the participants, the supervisors decided to pursue the formulation of minimal goals for expected student achievement in certain competency areas. The pertinent areas were identified, then assigned to paired individuals for the drafting of goals via collaborative effort. Ensuing seminar meetings were devoted to the authors' presentations of their goals and to appropriate group discussion. In this manner, broad achievement goals were constructed for each of three proficiency levels: beginning, intermediate, and advanced. This framework not only provided necessary structure and direction for the participants, but also resulted in an applicable set of guidelines for use with students, as shown in Appendix VI.

The availability of established goals has prompted the group to examine the next logical topic, student evaluation. Several fundamental questions have been addressed: How can the supervisor know when goals have been reached? Should priorities be set for certain competencies? How does goal-attainment translate into an equitable grading system? These matters have yet to be resolved. And so our quest for answers in audiology supervision continues to be the recurrent seminar theme.

Supervision has taken its rightful, and apparently permanent, place in our continuing education work. (It is assumed that supervisors will continue to keep abreast of current developments in clinical audiology; any continuing education effort should concern itself with this important need.) If our experimental endeavors at Northwestern University have predictability, the potential benefits of this kind of program are many. Surely, they can be grouped into two major categories: (1) a fertile source for research ideas on supervision in audiology; and (2) a means for the improvement of supervisors' morale, as well as the quality of supervision.

SUPERVISION PRACTICUM FOR SUPERVISORS IN TRAINING

In keeping with Schubert's minimum requirement of "200 hours (internship) of practicum in supervision under the direction of a certified and experienced supervisor" (1974, p. 305), such an approach was inaugurated in the training of three new on-campus supervisors. At the start of each undertaking, these individuals were in various stages of their postgraduate careers: two had completed their Clinical Fellowship Year and received the Certificate of Clinical Competence in Audiology, and one was nearing this mark. Their years of clinical experience ranged in number from less than one to two complete years. Although these qualifications certainly fell short of the desired pre-supervision experience, all three participants were already on the staff, and we wanted and needed their supervisory services. Having compromised thusly, we were still hopeful that the development of a supervised supervision practicum system would partially offset the lack of clinical experience. At the very least, this would represent a significant improvement over the past method of preparing supervisors—no systematic preparation at all.

I assumed the role of supervising supervisor and proceeded in the following manner. The supervisors in training were first asked to read and digest some of the material that now comprises earlier chapters of this book. Afterward, two of the trainees acknowledged that they had already been familiar with many of the supervision techniques contained in this model, undoubtedly because they were products of our training program and had been supervised by me as students. Nonetheless, they reported, this required reading had given them new insight into the supervisory process and helped to organize their thoughts on preparation for the new role. The third trainee, a graduate from a different audiology program, found the reading even more beneficial.

During later staff schedulings of clinical practicum assignments, students at intermediate levels in their clinical work were selected for the trainees to supervise during the ensuing school quarter. Two students each were assigned to two of the trainees, and one student to the remaining trainee. And, in accordance with the previously described competency building plan for students, a parallel competency building schedule for supervisors in training was instituted. It was first implemented in these cases by assigning the participants to clinical activities involving the basic audiometric testing of adults. My contribution to the two-student arrangement was to monitor each trainee's supervision of one of his students quite closely throughout the quarter by way of observation, note taking, and postsession conferences, and to serve in an advisory capacity for the other weekly assignment with his second student. This two-fold alternating approach was designed purposely to give the trainees an opportunity to apply the first day's lessons to the second day's clinical activity, then air the second day's concerns during the following conference, and so on. Moreover, it would mutually serve the cross-purposes of thorough monitoring and complete independence, yet maintain consistency for the sake of the students. For the trainee having just one student, practicum was limited to the single weekly session with close surveillance.

Individual planning conferences were held with each trainee. Prior to the first clinical session, the supervisors in training were asked to prepare an outline of clinic orientation plans for the first student, a sort of lesson plan to guide them on that important first day. Because some of the students had not previously been assigned to clinical practicum duty in the medical school setting, it became important to talk about that clinic's idiosyncracies in detail, along with goals for the quarter. Preparation for this orientation gave the beginning supervisors a sense of security for their first student encounters. Furthermore, we had deliberately not scheduled a patient in the first appointment slot of the two- or three-patient assignments to allow ample time for familiarization of the students with medical charts and test equipment. In each instance, the beginning supervisor and I explained our separate and distinct roles to the participating student.

The supervised supervision sessions proceeded according to plan. During the initial first-day weekly sessions, I monitored the activities throughout each morning in order to get a complete picture of student-supervisor interactions, patient management, and supervisory competencies. After satisfying myself that certain requirements were being met, I opted to withdraw from the scene during the succeeding weeks for increasingly longer periods of time (depending on the complexity of the cases being seen), observing the workups of selected patients or selected tests for a given patient and, at times, simply spot checking the proceedings. Conferences were held with each new supervisor following all those sessions during which I took notes and/or made observations that warranted such discussion, or when the morning's events prompted questions from the trainee. Often, such questions were handled during the course of clinical activity.[2] In many instances, the trainee was given my notes following our discussion so that he could review them and make plans for the next practicum session. During the final days of the assignment, fulltime observation was resumed in order to check the new supervisor's progress in all the important competency areas.

A final conference was held to review the quarter's events and to discuss in detail my evaluation of each trainee's work. The evaluation form used for this purpose is shown in Appendix VII. As can be seen, much of its content and format were structured to conform with desirable supervisory characteristics as outlined in Chapter 3. Without disclosing the confidential details of these particular trainees' evaluations, I can report that the system worked well—the assignment of students in the manner previously described; the supervising supervisor's participation; and measurable progress of the supervisors in training. All participants appeared to benefit from this unprecedented training endeavor. And I have been pleased to discover that the entire process of supervising supervisors parallels closely that of student supervision. As might be expected, all of the aforementioned supervisory competencies and techniques were

---

[2] In the midst of this first quarter of supervisory work, the supervisors in training also participated in the aforementioned inservice training sessions for staff supervisors.

found to be applicable at this level. Hence, I found myself to be prepared adequately for the new role; this is not to say, of course, that each succeeding experience was without modification and refinement of approaches used.

Where suitable in terms of staff responsibilities, the second stage in this training procedure has been the assignment of the new supervisors to more basic audiometric testing in conjunction with an adult hearing aid selection activity. And, in subsequent quarters, supervisory work that includes audiologic evaluation and management of a pediatric population, and then special auditory testing, is being added. Students at various levels, both beginning and advanced, are mixed into the schedule. This adherence to a training sequence and its competency-building features, coupled with the trainees' accumulation of clinical experience, will, it is hoped, result in the desired end—thoroughly and systematically trained supervisors in audiology.

CONCLUSION

As the reader has probably surmised from the tenor of this account of training experiences, we are encouraged by the results of our efforts in all three areas. Each has the potential for productive experimentation and further development. Undoubtedly, however, there are totally different approaches to the training of audiology supervisors. This is where the challenge lies: we need to explore. It is hoped that other programs will come forth with their own ideas, whether tried and tested or just in a theoretical stage, so that supervision in audiology can move ahead.

CHAPTER 6

THE STATUS OF SUPERVISORS AND SUPERVISION: A Perspective

CONTENTS

Nor has the position of supervisor been given the prestige and recognition it deserves . . . particularly in the minds of those administrators in the university structure who are responsible for such decisions as salaries, rank, promotion, and tenure. (Anderson, 1973b, p. 5)

Quality supervision is demanding, taking a great deal of time and energy; therefore, little time is left for research and publication. . . . (Schubert, 1974, p. 305)

One of the issues in supervision which our profession must face . . . is the low status of clinical supervisors: lowest paid, often the least experience, little input into the academic program with no status, impact, or clout, especially in university settings. (Anderson, 1975)

The comments showed that the respondents believed that professional colleagues judged the role of the clinical supervisor to be inferior to that of the teaching faculty. (Schubert and Aitchison, 1975, p. 444)

One might infer from the above remarks that the status of supervisors and supervision is questionable at best, and one might be right. A broad view of the supervision situation reveals a disquieting reality: the status of the clinical supervisor today is not much better than it was when this issue was addressed in 1963 at the National Conference on Graduate Education in Speech Pathology and Audiology (Darley, 1963). Certainly, more statements of concern are heard and suggested remedies are being proposed, as evidenced in articles and convention papers on supervision. But rhetoric alone will not advance the supervisor's cause. Persistent followup action in a concerted effort by many individuals is needed if supervisors in the field want to change their lot. It is essential that supervisors promote themselves and the importance of their work.

In this chapter, the reader is asked to turn his attention away from audiology supervision per se and back to supervision in the entire field of communicative disorders.

AN EXAMINATION OF PROBLEMS AND SOLUTIONS

Where do the problems lie? And what can be done?

The foremost difficulty might be designated as a group identity crisis. Who are supervisors and what do they do? As already stated in Chapters 2 and 3, the answers to these questions are determined to a great extent by the nature of specific jobs and the settings in which they are performed. But this is part of the problem: despite such differences among supervisory roles, common denominators need to be found, ones that identify supervisors as a group and portray them as the essential commodity they are. At the very least, this singlemindedness in role definition would seem to be an attainable goal for each of the major supervisor groupings; for example, public school vs. university, speech and language pathology vs. audiology. Supervisors cannot hope to convince others of their worth without a united front. Given the field's history of semantic differences over occupational titles and job definitions, however, the identification task may not be easy. It is nonetheless a necessary prerequisite to any crusade for equitable group recognition.

As has already been stressed in an earlier chapter, a clinical teaching definition of supervision is favored by this author. It would seem that this definition, and this definition only, offers any hope of elevating the university supervisor's[1] status to a level on par with academic faculty counterparts. Of course, supervisors cannot claim a right to the title of clinical teacher unless they earn that right. It is therefore incumbent upon all university supervisors to commit themselves totally to the clinical teaching process. The longer casual supervision by even a few persons is tolerated, the more distant will be any goal of convincing others in the field that supervisors are genuine teachers. The logical means to establishing and enforcing teaching standards exist in compulsory minimum requirements that include training and continuing education stipulations, and then lead to some kind of certification.

Once it has been demonstrated conclusively that supervisors *are* teachers, there will be a need to convince colleagues that clinical teaching, though different from classroom teaching, is not inferior to it. In Schubert and Aitchison's profile questionnaire (1975), 78% of the responding supervisors believed their work to be equal in importance to that of (classroom) teachers. Yet, as reflected in the quotation at the beginning of this chapter, many of them added that their coworkers did not share this feeling of equality. Although not stated specifically in the

---

[1] The remainder of this discussion is directed exclusively to the problems of the university supervisor whose fulltime responsibilities entail supervision.

profile report, it is highly probable that these "professional colleagues" are primarily other speech and language pathologists and audiologists. This being the case, supervisors can hardly anticipate more sensitive recognition by high-level administrators (deans of schools, boards of trustees) who have not been trained in the area of communicative disorders, because between the supervisors and the administrators stand the academic colleagues in communicative disorders. It is they who interpret to the policy-makers what supervisors do. In short, it is they who have the bargaining power to improve supervisor's conditions. But they will not exercise this power unless, and until, it is proven that supervisors' contributions to clinical training programs warrant higher recognition. Even if a convincing case were presented on behalf of supervisors, such a move by nonsupervisors is not likely to be made without a push from some external force. ASHA regulations, for example, could mandate change if promulgated through ETB standards in tandem with required certification for supervisors. Whatever the approach to this serious problem, supervisors must heed a number of obstacles, as illustrated in the following pages.

The persons upon whom supervisors must rely to articulate their plight to administrators stand to lose the exclusiveness of what might be called hard-earned territorial rights: faculty appointments, professorial ranks, tenure eligibility. Even if supervisors have direct access to administrators, it is virtually inconceivable that such faculty members would not also be consulted. And, as alluded to earlier, even those academic faculty persons who privately pledge allegiance to supervisors may not choose to follow through with affirmative action on the supervisors' behalf for a variety of reasons.

There are some supervisors who do not believe in themselves or their work enough to be discontented with their lot. They either are satisfied with the status quo or would rather accept it than "rock the boat." Such attitudes of apathy and/or resignation can only stand in the way of supervisors who are interested in upgrading the status of all their peers. What are the possible reasons for complacency? The first, and seemingly most obvious, is that supervisors believe their work is, in fact, inferior to that of their coworkers. Yet, according to Schubert and Aitchison's data (1975), less than 11% of the respondents had such a low opinion of their supervisory roles. It should be remembered, however, that all of these respondents were not "pure" supervisors, a likely contaminant in this datum.

Another factor might be what Muma, Mann, and Trenholm identified as a "somewhat transient trend" (1976, p. 423) in training programs in speech pathology and audiology. They noted that the overwhelming majority of master's level (as well as doctoral level) participants in a questionnaire survey had worked in their current department settings 10 or fewer years. Indeed, 88% of those at the instructor/clinical supervisor level had worked less than five years in their departments. The authors speculated on possible causes of the transiency: the large number of women who leave the profession in favor of homemaking; attainment of a higher degree; and changing places of employment. If this is so, it is not difficult to understand why some supervisors want to remain uninvolved: their interest in supervision is more temporary than permanent, more superficial than committed, more job-oriented than career-oriented.

The clinic/research controversy and the "publish or perish" demands in universities are not likely to be viewed differently for the sake of supervisors who seek more recognition for their type of work. This means that if a *fulltime* supervisor is given a faculty appointment, his chances of being advanced to ranks higher than instructor, or being granted tenure, are slight. And, as Schubert (1974) has discussed, most persons who devote themselves to quality supervision will not find adequate time to fulfill research and publishing requirements. As supervisors who work in active clinics with full student loads are aware, untold hours are spent doing the necessary homework that goes with the job. Invariably, those supervisors who break away from the low-status mold are those who have been given fewer responsibilities involving direct supervision. Supervisors are thus faced with an unrelenting paradox: they are being told that the only avenue to more prestigious levels is the research/publication route; yet the supervision role itself, if performed competently, has built-in roadblocks that preclude or hamper research/publication.

Some individuals argue that most supervisors, even if given the time for research activities, are not capable of assuming such responsibility, particularly since the majority are at the master's level and thus not trained in research techniques. If this is a prevailing attitude, the field of communicative disorders is in trouble. It is often the master clinicians and supervisors who are in the best position to identify clinical problems and explore alternative solutions in the actual clinical setting. If these people are not being given the opportunity to investigate, and any competent clincan/supervisor must think of researchable questions almost daily, an inestimable amount of talent is being wasted. In his keynote address at the ASHA North Central Regional Conference, Minifie (1975) spoke to this issue, seeking to quash the myth that research belongs only in the laboratory, and urging that clinicians be allotted time for research. If one considers his exhortation in the present discussion, it can be seen that the exclusion of clinical supervisors from experimental endeavors (by time constraints and role definition) not only keeps these persons on the bottom rung of the academic ladder, but also robs our profession of an invaluable resource. Moreover, the students of these supervisors are liable to be shortchanged for several reasons: (1) the supervisor with no opportunity to satisfy his own clinical curiosity may lose the probative bent and zeal that are so necessary to invigorating supervision; (2) there is no "scientific clinician" model for the student to emulate (Minifie (1975) calls for the training of scientific clinicians as well as clinical scientists, avowing that the future of this profession is linked with the development of both types); and (3) the student is being taught, by implication, that the clinician waits for the researcher to develop clinically acceptable techniques.

It is interesting to ponder the fact that virtually all university clinicians are supervisors, this being the reason for their employment in such a setting in the first place. Universities do not customarily hire clinicians per se (that is, persons who see patients regularly but have no attendant supervisory responsibilities) to conduct patient-oriented research. Those individuals who are hired specifically to carry out prede-termined research projects on restricted clinical populations do not qualify for such a category because they engage in tightly designed research studies with all the natural variables under control, and then proceed to test their carefully selected subjects in a systematic manner. And most university persons who plan and oversee such research have little direct contact with patients on a daily basis because most of their time is consumed by administrative and academic responsibilities. As a consequence, the university person who has the greatest accessibility to the everyday patient, yet has the least opportunity to effect change through spontaneous clinical experimentation, is the supervisor.

A final consideration in this regard is the urgently needed research of the supervisory process itself. It is difficult to imagine that this responsibility would be handled by anyone other than practicing super-visors. Again, however, one cannot expect much to be accomplished unless sufficient time is set aside for these persons to contemplate their research objectives, study supervisory options, and design appropriate investigations, as well as analyze the results afterwards and prepare rele-vant information for publication. Even the most industrious supervisors are likely to find such productiveness unachievable unless they opt to sacrifice some of their more demanding, time-consuming obligations to students and patients. Compromises of this sort can only serve to weaken the quality of their regular supervision, thereby directly conflicting with the original intent of supervision research—the improvement of supervision. And so the busiest, and often the best, supervisors may avoid the plunge into supervision research out of sheer loyalty to their own supervision. And once again, the field is victimized.

There are other obstacles and consequences that may impede the supervisor's quest for status elevation, and they are even more elusive than those just presented. A sexism factor is often suggested, but is exceedingly difficult to prove, given the imbalance of male/female levels of degree attainment and related job assignments in the field. The preponderance of fulltime supervisory positions belongs to master's level females, a circumstance that most persons recognize as being a fact but one that has to be revealed through controlled investigation. Schubert and Aitchison's data (1975) approached this revelation, yet failed to isolate it per se (Shriberg et al., 1975b). This assumption might be considered along with the most recent report on personal income of ASHA members, which states: "it seems most appropriate to conclude that Members of the Association who are female receive substantially lower salaries than Members who are male regardless of their age, highest degree, or employment setting" (Curlee, 1975, p. 30). Because salaries are principally linked to rank and status within the university hierarchy, one must wonder how the latter contribute to the male/female discrepancy in salary statistics emanating from university settings. It would also be enlightening to determine the relationship of highest degree and number of years of professional experience with academic rank and job description, and then compare these data for males and females. None of the surveys cited herein has examined these important questions. Somewhere in the midst of such information lie answers to the sexism issue regarding supervisors.

Another possible deterrent to supervisors' pursuits of equitable treatment from colleagues and administrators might be found in the low-status stigma itself. That is to say, those persons in supervisory roles who have higher ambitions than such positions will allow them to satisfy may opt to seek a doctoral degree and move themselves into jobs with rank and opportunity for advancement. This falls into line with the aforementioned movement theory proposed by Muma, Mann, and Trenholm (1976). In making their move, these individuals are likely to abandon supervisory work, either wholly or partially, in favor of academic teaching and/or other occupational endeavors. This conceivable sequence of events gives rise to several unsettling questions. Are supervisory roles being used as steppingstones to more exalted positions? If so, are the individuals who pursue vertical movement doing so because they actually want to be something other than supervisors or because nonsupervisory roles promise better salaries and fringe benefits? To come to the point, is the field losing some of its best supervisors, or best potential supervisors, to other roles because of the status problem? And are those remaining to carry out the bulk of the supervisory load interested in raising their sights, or have the leaders moved on, leaving the followers behind? The answers to such questions, of course, would be largely speculative given the inadequate knowledge of individual motivations regarding career plans and the state of the art in evaluating supervisory effectiveness. Nonetheless, they touch on areas of potential concern because they may have a bearing on the types of persons who supervise, the number of persons who remain committed to fulltime supervision for the duration of their professional careers, and the resultant efficacy of those who strive to upgrade the status of supervisors.

A STUDY AND SOME CONCLUSIONS

When difficulties with the supervisor recognition problem were experienced in our own institution, other university training programs in speech pathology and audiology were queried regarding their current appointment procedures for supervisors. Brief questionnaires were sent to member universities of the Midwest Big-Ten Conference.[2] Eight of the nine contacts responded, thereby giving us a total sample of nine programs after adding our own input. The results were both fascinating and puzzling: we found that nearly all of these programs deal with their supervisors differently. Indeed, there probably could have been no greater diversity in such a small sample.

The programs were questioned about the status of their fulltime supervisors only. This automatically eliminated one program that utilizes its academic faculty members to fulfill supervisory roles in addition to their other duties. Interestingly, this respondent was the only one who made it a point to identify supervising as clinical teaching. Another program also reported that academic faculty members are involved in clinical supervision, but that this is supplemented by fulltime clinical supervisors, all having faculty appointments. Of the latter, all but one person (an assistant professor in a tenure track) are on the instructor level with temporary one-year appointments.

Two programs divide their supervisors into faculty appointment and professional staff (nonfaculty) categories. In the first of these, one supervisor has a faculty appointment as assistant professor and has been

---

[2] In addition to Northwestern University, this includes the University of Illinois, Indiana University, University of Iowa, the University of Michigan, Michigan State University, the University of Minnesota, Ohio State University, Purdue University, and the University of Wisconsin. The survey was conducted during the summer of 1976.

granted tenure, whereas the remaining supervisors have professional staff status with no attendant tenure eligibility. The other program with a two-level approach has given faculty appointments to some of its fulltime supervisors, while others are on the professional staff. All of these with faculty status, however, are normally placed in a non-tenure track, having been assigned special non-tenured ranks. Some of these appointments have multiple-year contracts. Tenure is available only to those who elect to pursue the regular academic ranking system with its research/publication requirements.

Faculty appointments for all fulltime supervisors are reportedly given in two of the responding programs. In one of these, the supervisors are still at the instructor level with no opportunity to advance in rank, yet have been placed in a tenure track. The second program in this category has placed all its supervisors in a tenure track—several instructors, an assistant professor, and an associate professor. Two of these supervisors (apparently the latter two) have already been granted tenure.

Finally, in contrast to those programs just described, three respondents in this survey reported that none of their fulltime supervisors has a faculty appointment. Instead, all have professional staff status with no tenure in the offing. One of the programs has given these persons the professional staff title of specialist, a staff position available in that particular university.

Whether or not this sampling represents a microcosm of the university training programs in this country, it strikingly reveals the different ways in which supervisory positions are viewed and handled. The rationale behind all these variations is unknown, of course. One can only surmise that certain obstacles, such as those presented earlier in this discussion, are more operative at some universities than at others. Be that as it may, the inconsistency is no less disturbing. Our profession must take steps to acknowledge that there are, in fact, many differences of opinion, and then seek to reconcile them through studied debate. It should go without saying that supervisors ought to be included in any deliberation.[3] This should be followed by the establishment of firm guidelines and perhaps the eventual adoption of ASHA-enforced regulations as suggested before. The ASHA Committee on Supervision in Speech Pathology and Audiology can lead the way. The quality of supervision, training programs, and training program graduates all depends on the outcome of this overdue proceeding.

---

[3] Supervisors can begin helping themselves by joining the Council of University Supervisors of Practicum in Speech Pathology and Audiology.

As indicated herein, many questions will need to be resolved. The crux of the issue is straightforward: should clinical teaching (supervision) be regarded as an equivalent counterpart of academic teaching? In considering the answer to this pivotal question, decisions will need to be made about the nature of supervision that transpires in university training programs. Is supervision being done at varying levels of sophistication that warrant different types of appointments for supervisors? Or is all clinical supervision in the university setting essentially the same, thereby calling for equal recognition of everyone in this role, with the only variables being years of service in the institution and academic degree? How does merit fit into this consideration, and how can this be assessed? Is there an acceptable way to evaluate the performance of supervisors? If it is determined that clinical teaching is not commensurate with academic teaching but is still worthy of faculty status, the rank and tenure issues will need to be addressed. Is it possible, for example, to establish a system of clinical ranks that parallels the traditional academic ranking system?[4] And could such a system embrace a tenure track that has criteria other than research and publication output? Or should the latter requirements be retained with the stipulation that supervisory positions allow time for the pursuit of such endeavors? These are but a few of the questions that need to be asked and answered.

The job will be difficult but it must be done. Despite the transience of supervisory personnel, our field and its training programs are now old enough to have a sizeable number of supervisors who have accumulated more than a few years of creditable professional work experience in their roles. These people must be recognized for the contributions they have made to the training of speech pathologists and audiologists. And, at the same time, clinical supervision must be sufficiently rewarding to attract, and keep, knowledgeable, forward-looking individuals who will add to its impact on our profession.

EPILOGUE

Not wishing to end this presentation on a disheartening note, I can report that the rewards of university-oriented clinical supervision are fortunately not limited to faculty appointments, salaries, tenure, and professional rights. As every clinician knows, helping patients is immeasurably rewarding. In addition to this source of gratification, the

---

[4] An exemplary model has been developed at the University of Connecticut (Ulrich and Giolas, 1977).

clinical supervisor stands to be rewarded by the accomplishments of his students. To watch a student progress from a helpless state of unenlightenment to a level of clinical expertise, knowing that the supervised clinical practicum contributed greatly to that growth, can be even more gratifying because the supervisor has that much more investment of time, energy, and self in the end product. And to see a graduate earn the praise of others in his chosen work or achieve a mark of distinction in this field is the contributing supervisor's ultimate reward, a reward that defies description.

APPENDICES

APPENDIX I

EVALUATION OF STUDENT IN CLINICAL PRACTICUM

This is a sample of the student clinician evaluation form currently used in Northwestern University's audiology program. The first sections on professionalism were designed to mutually serve students in other related clinical areas. (This entire form is currently under review by Northwestern University supervisors in their seminar deliberations on student evaluation.)

Student _____ Supervisor _____ Date _____

Clinic Site _____ Type of Assignment _____

Quarter_____ Quarter of work in clinic (1st, 2d, etc.) _____

Rate the student's professional competencies in terms of the following scale by circling the most appropriate number:

1. *Unsatisfactory*—means awareness of competency not apparent
2. *Fair*—means awareness of competency apparent but not implemented
3. *Average*—means competency demonstrated 50% of the time
4. *Good*—means competency demonstrated 75% of the time
5. *Excellent*—means competency demonstrated consistently

If you are unable to rate an item or it is not appropriate, circle "X" for the item.

PROFESSIONAL RESPONSIBILITY

		Unsatis-factory	Fair	Average	Good	Excellent	Unable to rate or not appropriate
1.	Punctuality in reporting to assignment	1	2	3	4	5	X
2.	Promptness in submitting written plans/reports/summaries	1	2	3	4	5	X
3.	Orderliness in maintaining clinic room/test suite/equipment	1	2	3	4	5	X
4.	Attendance and participation in group and individual supervision sessions	1	2	3	4	5	X
5.	Demonstration of initiative	1	2	3	4	5	X

Comments_____

PROFESSIONAL INTERACTION

		Unsatis-factory	Fair	Average	Good	Excellent	Unable to rate or not appropriate
1.	Approachability and responsiveness to supervisor	1	2	3	4	5	X
2.	Approachability and responsiveness to students/patients	1	2	3	4	5	X
3.	Respect for students/patients	1	2	3	4	5	X
4.	Effectiveness in dealing with parents	1	2	3	4	5	X
5.	Poise in professional interactions	1	2	3	4	5	X

Comments_____

PROFESSIONAL ATTITUDE/BEHAVIOR

		Unsatis-factory	Fair	Average	Good	Excellent	Unable to rate or not appropriate
1.	Pride in professional role	1	2	3	4	5	X
2.	Interest in clinical assignment	1	2	3	4	5	X
3.	Interest in improving performance	1	2	3	4	5	X
4.	Emotional control and stability	1	2	3	4	5	X
5.	Attainment of self-evaluation skills	1	2	3	4	5	X

Comments_____

FOR STUDENTS IN AUDIOLOGY

KNOWLEDGE AND APPLICATION OF TEST TECHNIQUES

Rate the student's knowledge of test techniques and his competence in applying this knowledge in clinical work in terms of the following scale:

1. Unsatisfactory—means cannot or will not learn techniques; needs constant supervision.
2. Fair—means slow to learn; responds poorly to teaching; needs supervision on most tasks.
3. Average—means knows test techniques fairly well; requires moderate amount of supervision.

4. Good—means well informed on most aspects of testing; seldom requires assistance.
5. Excellent—means completely knowledgeable on all phases of testing; works independently.

If you are unable to rate an item or it is not appropriate, circle "X" for the item.

Conventional audiometry

		Unsatis-factory	Fair	Average	Good	Excellent	Unable to rate or not appropriate
1.	Giving instructions	1	2	3	4	5	X
2.	Air conduction techniques	1	2	3	4	5	X
3.	Bone conduction techniques	1	2	3	4	5	X
4.	Speech audiometric techniques	1	2	3	4	5	X
5.	Use of masking	1	2	3	4	5	X
6.	Impedance audiometry	1	2	3	4	5	X

Comments_____

Pediatric audiometry

		Unsatis-factory	Fair	Average	Good	Excellent	Unable to rate or not appropriate
1.	Behavior-shaping and management of child	1	2	3	4	5	X
2.	Play audiometry	1	2	3	4	5	X
3.	VRA	1	2	3	4	5	X
4.	TROCA	1	2	3	4	5	X
5.	Warble tone audiometry	1	2	3	4	5	X
6.	Speech audiometric techniques	1	2	3	4	5	X

Comments_____

Hearing aid selection (Check: Adults____ Children____)

		Unsatis-factory	Fair	Average	Good	Excellent	Unable to rate or not appropriate
1.	Determination of amplification options	1	2	3	4	5	X
2.	Selection of individual hearing aids, instrument settings, and earmold types	1	2	3	4	5	X
3.	Subjective evaluation skills	1	2	3	4	5	X
4.	Earmold fitting, volume setting skills	1	2	3	4	5	X

	Unsatis-factory	Fair	Average	Good	Excellent	Unable to rate or not appropriate
5. Trouble-shooting skills	1	2	3	4	5	X
6. Selection of appropriate tests	1	2	3	4	5	X
7. Interpretation of subjective and objective findings, and attendant decision making	1	2	3	4	5	X

Comments_____

Special auditory tests

	Unsatis-factory	Fair	Average	Good	Excellent	Unable to rate or not appropriate
1. Instructions	1	2	3	4	5	X
2. Administration	1	2	3	4	5	X
3. Selection of appropriate tests	1	2	3	4	5	X
4. Interpretation of individual tests	1	2	3	4	5	X
5. Interpretation of test profile	1	2	3	4	5	X
6. Insight regarding significance of individual test results as well as test profile	1	2	3	4	5	X

Comments_____

OTHER CLINICAL ACTIVITIES

Rate the student's competency in handling nontest clinical activities in terms of the following scale:

1. Unsatisfactory—means work unacceptable; always must be redone.
2. Fair—means work barely passable; often must be redone.
3. Average—means average quality; moderate number of inadequacies present, but improvement evident.
4. Good—means work of good quality; few inadequacies.
5. Excellent—means work always excellent; almost no need for supervisory monitoring/correction.

If you are unable to rate an item or it is not appropriate, circle "X" for the item.

	Unsatis-factory	Fair	Average	Good	Excellent	Unable to rate or not appropriate
Record keeping	1	2	3	4	5	X

Comments_____

	Unsatis-factory	Fair	Average	Good	Excellent	Unable to rate of not appropriate
Resumé writing	1	2	3	4	5	X

Comments_____

	Unsatis-factory	Fair	Average	Good	Excellent	Unable to rate or not appropriate
Report writing	1	2	3	4	5	X

Comments_____

	Unsatis-factory	Fair	Average	Good	Excellent	Unable to rate or not appropriate
History taking	1	2	3	4	5	X

Comments_____

	Unsatis-factory	Fair	Average	Good	Excellent	Unable to rate or not appropriate
Knowledge and appropriate utilization of terminology	1	2	3	4	5	X

Comments_____

	Unsatis-factory	Fair	Average	Good	Excellent	Unable to rate or not appropriate
Evaluation review with patient/family						
Level of student participation:						
1. Feedback on test findings	1	2	3	4	5	X
2. Rehabilitative counseling	1	2	3	4	5	X

Comments_____

	Unsatis-factory	Fair	Average	Good	Excellent	Unable to rate or not appropriate
Checking test equipment						
1. Listening check of pure tone audiometer and masker prior to use	1	2	3	4	5	X
2. Detection of problems in audiometer or masker	1	2	3	4	5	X
3. Cleaning and demag-netization of tape recorder	1	2	3	4	5	X
4. Listening check of speech audiometer for speech signal via earphone and loudspeaker, and masking signal via earphone and loudspeaker	1	2	3	4	5	X
5. Detection of problems in tape recorder and speech audiometer	1	2	3	4	5	X
6. Calibration of pure tone audiometer and speech audiometer	1	2	3	4	5	X
7. Interpretation and appli-cation of calibration data	1	2	3	4	5	X

Comments_____

GENERAL COMMENTS

In the space below, make any additional comments you feel are important regarding the student's performance in this clinical assignment:

Midterm Report_____

Final Report_____   CLINICAL GRADE_____

_____	_____	_____	_____
Date	Student (signature)	Date	Supervisor (signature)

APPENDIX II

GUIDE TO TAPED SUPERVISION SESSIONS

In the audiology supervision course for students at Northwestern University, one of the projects for out-of-class completion assigns students to listen to four and one-half hours of audiotaped supervision sessions, using accompanying printed guides and copies of related patient records. The taped material represents various kinds of supervisory activities, and excerpts are shown here, describing in detail: clinical activity; physical setting/location of participants; patient code; clinical competency being taught; level of participating student; and a step-by-step account of the taped supervision process.

STUDENT 1 (1st year, 1st quarter, 3d week in clinic)

Listening Check of Equipment

Time: 8 Minutes

Setting Supervisor operating equipment, student listening. (1st week, no listening check was done; 2d week, supervisor had operated equipment while student listened—thus, this taped sequence represents student's second exposure to this process.)

Method
A. Reviewed plan of action before beginning.
B. Repeated steps throughout listening check as they were carried out.
C. Asked student to explain what had been done, and the reasons for doing it after she had been told several minutes previously. This was done to determine whether or not she understood the rationale for the procedure— i.e., was further explanation necessary at this point?—and to find out how much of the procedure she could remember after having been told twice (once on this date, and once the week before). The latter helped me to know if she was ready to operate the equipment by herself during the listening check the following week; I determined that she indeed was ready, and the performance the next week proved this to be true.
D. Explored with student the possible reasons for defect in equipment in order to make her think about these possibilities. This should help her to understand the equipment better and prepare her for future trouble-shooting occurrences. (The source of the equipment problem described here was indeed in the audiometer itself, and was subsequently solved through repair.)
E. Praised student for having detected problem.

Excerpted for this publication. Key to abbreviations: AA—basic audiometric assessment for adult patients; AE—audiologic evaluation (AA plus sound field speech audiometry); SHA—selection of hearing aid; HAE—AE/SHA combination; h/a—hearing aid.

Comments   The listening check procedure described here is more extensive than may be required on a daily basis, but it serves several instructive purposes:

A. Makes the student aware of the number of potential equipment problems and how they might be identified.
B. Encourages good listening habits. (After student has been thoroughly familiarized with both roles in the listening check procedure, this is usually alternated from week to week, i.e., he may sometimes be asked to listen, other times to operate the equipment.)
C. Forces the student to operate the equipment quickly and, eventually, without hesitation.

Review of Patient's Medical Chart and Preparation for Interview
Time: 17 Minutes   (Patient A)

Setting   AA assignment. Review of medical chart with student, while preparing her for her first patient interview. (1st week she was not required to participate at all in this task; 2d week was her first attempt at interpreting, summarizing and recording medical chart information—but only through collaboration with supervisor, as demonstrated in this taped sequence.)

Method
A. Otologic report reviewed word by word with student.
B. Interpretation of medical symbols and terminology provided for student.
C. Periodic questions asked of student to determine her level of understanding in certain areas. Clarification given where deemed appropriate. Much of this carried out to determine how much she remembered from the previous week, and to assess her progress in this area, i.e., when do I think she will be ready to take on this task more independently?
D. Gradual transition made from discussion of otologic findings to preparation for interview:
    1. Discussion of history form with student, and of how to incorporate medical information into the structure of this form.
    2. Discussion of possible reasons behind certain otologic findings, how they might relate to one another (e.g., physical findings vs. tuning fork test results), and how they might help us to speculate on the type of hearing problem we are about to encounter. This discussion helps to introduce the student to integration of otologic and audiologic concepts, and their application to an actual clinical case.
E. Student given suggestions on how to ask specific questions, how to deal with various answers, and how to probe for additional information when indicated by certain patient answers. (This was also done during the previous week's medical chart reviews, but with the understanding that I would be conducting the interview.)
F. Student given assurance that if patient gives information in area with which student is unfamiliar (in this case, hearing aid history), I would take over.
G. Student asked if she felt she was ready to conduct patient interview on her own. If she had responded negatively, I would have accepted this and proceeded to do the interview myself.
    Note: The fact that she accepted this first-interview assignment, knowing that she was going to be recorded, is a rather obvious indicator of her self-confidence and readiness for the task.

Patient Interview
Time: 5 Minutes

Setting   Student conducted interview while I sat in control room listening.

Postinterview Discussion
Time: 4 Minutes

Method
A.   Reviewed aloud the student's recorded information, adding suggestions where appropriate and reinforcing those points that needed emphasis, e.g., in this case:
   1.   Use of appropriate terminology in recording information.
   2.   Importance of not allowing the form itself to dictate questioning sequence.
B.   Praised student on overall good job. (This is not necessary every time, but is certainly indicated in this instance because she had never taken a history before. Even though neither the questioning nor the recording aspects of her history-taking were perfect, the use of praise at this point was indicated because (1) she actually did do a good job for her first try, and (2) the praise will instill more self-confidence in her—which is extremely important at this stage.)

Preparation for Giving Instructions (Pure Tone)
Time: 3 Minutes

Method
A.   Student asked to recite sample instructions to supervisor. (This was previously discussed with her during her first two clinic sessions, but she had done it by herself with several patients only during the second such session, thus only on one day before.)
B.   Suggestions given for improvement—and the reasons for them.
C.   Rather unrelated comment about degree of hearing loss expected, but this should be done at this point because it had already been discussed with her during the preparation for her interview, and now, after having talked with the patient, she should be able to draw some sort of tentative conclusion in this regard. Thus, this discussion completes the question that had been considered earlier—and provides the student with some reasonable expectations about the hearing test results.

Test Instructions, Earphone Placement, Postinstructions Discussion
Time: 2 Minutes

Setting   Student giving instructions while I remained outside test room listening.

Method
A.   After student gave instructions, I joined her in test room to be sure earphone placement was correct, by watching her and giving suggestions. (She had already done this the previous week, but had not done it enough times yet for me to feel completely assured that she was doing it correctly on

her own. Even for the more experienced student, this should be checked periodically. Right vs. left should be consistently checked by supervisor!)
B.   After leaving test room with student, reinforced some critical points in her test instructions.

Pure Tone Testing: Air Conduction, Bone Conduction, Bone Conduction with Masking
Time: 16 Minutes

Method
A.   Air conduction testing:
    1.   Discussed the following areas with student during course of testing:
        a.   Setting up equipment.
        b.   Which ear to start testing.
        c.   Starting level.
        d.   Threshold pursuit. (Details of this discussed in previous weeks, thus not necessary at this stage.)
        e.   Consistency of patient's responses.
    2.   After testing completed:
        Discussion of degree of loss—possible reason for its lack of agreement with our earlier expectations. (Excellent observations given by student here.)
B.   Bone conduction testing:
    1.   Before testing (still in control room with student):
        a.   Which ear to start testing.
        b.   Need for masking?
        c.   Review of test instructions for bone conduction testing; student asked to give sample instructions to supervisor first.
    2.   Entered test room with student to observe bone conduction oscillator placement, make suggestions, and demonstrate.
    3.   During testing:
        a.   Discussion of threshold pursuit.
        b.   Starting level.
        c.   Recording symbols.
    4.   Following testing on one ear (mastoid):
        Need for further bone conduction testing and possibility of using masking.
C.   Bone conduction testing with masking:
    1.   Before testing (still in control room):
        a.   How to set up earphones and bone oscillator for masking, i.e., right vs. left, etc.
        b.   Review masking instructions, asking student to say them to supervisor first.
    2.   Masking instructions given by student, while I remained outside test room.
    3.   Entered test room to demonstrate/observe earphone and bone conduction oscillator placement, and make suggestions.
    4.   During testing:
        a.   Review setup of equipment.
        b.   Procedural discussion:
            1.   Need to determine unmasked threshold?
            2.   Amount of masking needed, interaural attenuation.

3. Starting level for tone presentation.
4. Occlusion effect due to earphone placement.
5. Hood technique, step by step.
6. Recording threshold, masking amount.

Patient Interview with Supervisor Also Participating, Earphone Placement, Pure Tone Test Instructions. Postinterview Discussion

Time: 14 Minutes   (Patient C)

Method

A. Interview initiated by student, but I entered room shortly after she began. (This interview was preceded by some prestructuring—*not recorded*—at time of medical chart review.) This, then, is an example of how a supervisor can participate along with a beginning student during the course of a patient interview, and how such intervention can be used for instructive purposes. In this case I deemed intervention to be warranted and appropriate for several reasons:

1. The history was sufficiently complex that the student needed some structuring and guidance that could not have been given to her before the patient was seen, as I could not possibly have known in advance what the patient's replies to certain questions would be.
2. The student was too inexperienced at this point to carry out such an interview completely on her own. On the other hand, she was prepared to ask *some* of the questions by herself. Thus, there is a choice for the supervisor to take in this situation, i.e., something between having the student do the interview on her own vs. the supervisor conducting the interview as the student listens. (Although listening to the supervisor is a good experience, active student participation is better.)
3. The patient in this instance was obviously not inhibited or disturbed by my interaction with the student during the interview. Some patients, of course, might be disturbed by the obvious instruction time which is being taken at their expense; thus, the supervisor must be cautious about using this method in the presence of certain patients. If a problem is anticipated, particularly during supervision of beginning students, the supervisor must opt in the patient's favor by either conducting the interview herself or letting the student do it, then following this with her own questions later during the evaluation. If the latter course is chosen, I feel it's better not to do the additional questioning immediately following the student's interview because the patient will undoubtedly pick up the idea that the student's questioning was inadequate.
4. Point-by-point discussion during the interview is obviously more meaningful to the student than is postinterview instruction. Even though it may seem to be disruptive, my experience is that the student retains better what he has been told at the time he is doing it.

B. After interview:
1. Earphone placement.
   Still in test room with student and patient, I reminded student to ask patient to remove glasses and earrings. (Even though student may have encountered this before, I could not be completely certain, because it's difficult for me to remember exactly which student I've told what in previous weeks; thus, when in doubt, it's simply better to tell a student something—if he's heard it before, it will just serve as a reinforcement

and, if not, the supervisor will not have to send the student back into the test room to redo something, as might have happened here.)

2. Test instructions
    Knowing student was now capable of giving test instructions independently, I left the test room. My absence from the scene also possibly served another purpose here: if the patient had, in fact, inwardly questioned the student's competence during our two-person interview—which I seriously doubt in this case—the student's instructions, given independently and fairly smoothly, would be reassuring to the patient.

C. Postinterview discussion (back in control room with student just prior to testing):
    1. Explanation to student of why I took part in what had initially been intended to be her exclusive job. As mentioned before, I had not anticipated stepping in until I actually heard the patient's replies—but all my students are told not to be surprised if I do intervene in any part of a test situation. The important point here is that the student be told by the supervisor why she is entering into the situation.
    2. Need for structuring history is stressed to student, and how this need is perfectly illustrated in this particular case is pointed out.

STUDENT 2   (2d year, 4th quarter in clinic, 3d week in this SHA assignment with me. 1 previous AE/SHA assignment with a different supervisor)

Preparation for SHA Case

Time: 17 Minutes   (Patient D)

Method

A. Discussion of background information on case as reported in AA resumé.
    Selected those points that would determine our approach to SHA:
    1. Review of patient's hearing aid history and its implications. (Questioned student here on what factors she felt might have contributed to patient's poor performance with hearing aid during AA measurement.)
    2. Need for retesting performance with own aid and rationale for this.
    3. Patient's motivation for buying a new aid.
    4. Subjective vs. objective findings in h/a selection on a patient with severe hearing loss and discrimination problem.
    5. Kinds of instruments to choose for testing (student asked for suggestions):
        a. Gain?—Frequency response?—Compression amplification?
        b. Advisable to obtain unaided SRT?
    6. What should be done first?
        a. Find out age of aid from patient.
        b. Do listening check of patient's aid.
        c. Check manufacturers' specifications for patient's aid.

B. With student, had time to check specifications on patient's aid before he arrived. Discussed accordingly:
    1. Meaning of specifications, and how they relate to patient's hearing loss.
    2. Speculation on appropriateness of patient's own aid.

C. Discussion of test materials to be used:
    1. The need for selected spondees and how to select them.
    2. Need to use earphones for refamiliarizing patient with spondees.

Supplemental History-taking, Listening Check of Patient's Aid, Specs
Instruction, Preparation for Testing

Time: 12 Minutes

Method

A. Student questioned patient about age of hearing aid (unrecorded). I then entered the test room with patient and student.
B. While student was checking battery and performing listening check on patient's aid, I proceeded to ask patient some additional questions—for several reasons:
    1. I felt we needed more information that had not been discussed.
    2. The student could hear what questions I was asking and how I attempted to communicate with the patient.
    3. We could save time by acting as a team and doing two activities simultaneously (i.e., listening check and supplemental history).
    4. I could get an idea about the patient's unaided communicative efficiency as well as his perception of his difficulties with h/a use.
C. Additional information sought:
    1. Where was h/a purchased?
    2. Had the h/a been checked by the dealer and had it required repair?
D. I then checked with student regarding the results of her listening check. The only way I could determine whether or not her conclusions were well founded was to listen to the aid myself. Because there was some disagreement, I took the opportunity to discuss what we should be listening for, and the reasons for my conclusions:
    1. Internal noise.
    2. Loudness of aid relative to volume setting.
    3. Clarity of aid.
    Following this discussion, I had the student listen to the aid again—to demonstrate to her the points I had just covered.
E. I then discussed with student the supplemental history information I had just obtained from the patient, and the possible implications of this additional information.
F. Reviewed specifications again relative to patient's aid.
G. Checked earmold and discussed possible reasons for mold being vented.
H. Summarized points of listening check and how they might affect our final recommendation, pending test results.
I. Discussion of spondees to be used. (Student then refamiliarized patient with spondees—unrecorded.)
J. Discussion of need to know where h/a volume set by patient:
    1. Discussed this with patient and also checked the setting myself.
    2. Asked patient if aid is normally loud enough.
    3. Discussed the implications of these findings with student.
K. Decision made to give patient list of four test spondees.

Hearing Aid Selection Procedure

Time: 31 Minutes

Method

A. Testing performance with patient's own aid (in control room with student):
    1. Advised student to present all four spondees at suprathreshold level to be sure patient could understand them through hearing aid.

    2.   Student established SRT (unrecorded).
    3.   Discussion of SRT and what it means in terms of gain being provided by aid.
    4.   Decision to use picture identification task for discrimination testing.
    5.   Choice of presentation level.
    6.   How best to administer test.
    7.   Student administered test (most of it unrecorded).
    8.   Decision to stop after ten words.
    9.   Decision to change to 60 dB HL presentation level and why.
  10.   Student administered test (unrecorded).
  11.   Discussed implications of better discrimination at 60 HL than at 50 HL, i.e., as indication to try on more powerful aids.

B.   After test—I discussed with patient his preference for eyeglass vs. BTE aid. (Now back in test room.)

C.   Discussion with student regarding choice of next aid to be tried:
    1.   Choice of brand.
    2.   Eyeglass (based on patient preference).
    3.   Gain.
    4.   Looked at specifications with student:
       a.   HAIC gain and output.
       b.   Forward mike.
       c.   Telephone switch—probably no need for this and why.
       d.   Frequency response.
       e.   Compression amplification (no tolerance problem yet evident).
    5.   Use patient's own mold.
    6.   Choice of battery.
    7.   Demonstrated to student how to set up aid.
    8.   Explained why decision of eyeglass vs. BTE instrument necessary at this time.
    9.   Use of patient's own tubing.
  10.   Explained how to achieve proper tone setting, then while student did this,
  11.   I filled in h/a worksheet.

D.   Student spoke to patient for informal evaluation to find out how it sounded. (She put aid on patient.)
    1.   I gave student suggestions on how this might be improved.
    2.   I then talked to patient, asking him to compare sound quality of this aid to that of his own. His favorable reply encouraged us to proceed with testing of his performance with this instrument.
   I asked student to give test instructions again.

E.   Testing of performance with second aid (back in control room again). Discussion with student:
    1.   Reminded student of importance of giving test instructions face to face.
    2.   Discussed patient's favorable response to aid.
    3.   Asked student what volume setting she had used.
    4.   Student established SRT.
    5.   Discussed implications of better SRT.
    6.   Student obtained discrimination score at 50 HL.
    7.   Discussed better discrimination score with this aid.

F.   After test (back in test room with patient and student):

    1.   Student obtained patient's posttest subjective reaction to this aid.

    2.   I added to her questions by asking patient how this instrument compared to his listening experiences with other instruments he had worn over the years.

    3.   Discussed the implications of this response and how this might indicate what aid should be tried next.

G. Next aid selected. With help of specifications, determined with student choice of gain and frequency response. Determined that there was no need to do formal testing with this instrument because informal evaluation in test room with patient was unsuccessful.

H. Choice of next aid—with student:

    1.   Discussed point that patient did not appear to have a significant tolerance problem, hence no apparent need to explore compression amplification.

    2.   Summarized results of last aid and how they might help us to know what to choose for next aid.

    3.   Response (tone setting) decided on basis of specifications.

I. Testing of performance with aid (back in control room with student):

    1.   Student established SRT.

    2.   Discussed implications of SRT—indicating no need for further testing with this instrument.

J. What to do next?

    1.   Recommended administration of Utley Lipreading Test with best clinic aid vs. patient's own aid—and what these results should help us to determine.

    2.   Student administered Utley Test under planned conditions. (She gave instructions, put aids on and took them off, while I sat in control room and observed.)

    3.   Advised student again to get patient's impression of comparative sound quality of these two instruments:

        a.   Student initiated this discussion with patient.

        b.   I then went into test room and asked patient how he felt about purchasing the favored aid. Patient responded by stating that he would rather have his own aid adjusted than invest more money in a new instrument.

        c.   Thus, we reviewed specifications and decided that this was a possibility.

        d.   I discussed this with patient, also telling him to have the earmold and the aid checked by the dealer regardless of whether or not the power of the aid could be adjusted.

K. Postevaluation/precounseling discussion (back in control room with student):

    1.   Discussed importance of patient's remarks in making final decision regarding recommendations.

    2.   Asked student if she would like to do the counseling.

    3.   Because she indicated that she would rather not do so in this case, I discussed with her what my approach would be in counseling the patient and the specific recommendations I planned to outline for the patient.

    4.   Discussed the reason for not having tested aided discrimination in noise or tolerance for loud sounds.

STUDENT 3   (2d year, 4th quarter in clinic, 4th week in this HAE assignment. 1 previous HAE assignment with a different supervisor)

Counseling by Student for HAE, Postcounseling Session

Time: 34 Minutes   (Patient F)

Setting   Sample of counseling session with deaf adult. (Precounseling suggestions not recorded.)

Method
Student unaware of being taped.
A.   Student counseling patient while I observed/listened in control room. At certain times, I made suggestions to student via loudspeaker in test room; this technique, of course, would not be advisable if a lengthy conversation is anticipated or if the supervisor feels it will bother the patient. If such is the case, it's much better for the supervisor to enter the test room, either during the counseling if necessary, or preferably at the end of the student's counseling, to make additional remarks.
Told student he had been taped, and that postcounseling discussion would be taped.
B.   Postcounseling discussion with student after patient had gone. Made several suggestions:
  1.   More frequent questioning of patient to find out what she was or was not comprehending.
  2.   Using normal hearing as base of reference on audiogram. Example of how to state this to patient given.
  3.   Need to simplify terminology more—in terms of both vocabulary difficulty and ease of lipreading.
  4.   More use of visual aids when introducing new concept to patient, as recommendation card.
  (Note: Tape ran out here, so following was not recorded:)
  5.   Counseling should have been much more concise and to the point.
  6.   Explanation of test results was too detailed and too abstract.
  7.   Should have placed more emphasis on the limitations of amplification for a profound loss.

STUDENT 4   (2d year, 4th quarter in clinic, 10th week in this SHA assignment with me.)

Counseling by Student for SHA, Postcounseling Session

Time: 29 Minutes   (Patient G)

Setting   Sample of counseling session. (Precounseling suggestions not recorded.)

Method
Student unaware of being taped.
A.   Student counseling patient while I observed/listened in control room. I made several comments to student via loudspeaker from control room—primarily when patient asked questions to which she did not know the answers. One important correction I failed to make: dealer does not refund all money at conclusion of trial rental period if patient returns aid!

Told student she had been taped, and that postcounseling discussion would be taped.

B. Postcounseling discussion with student after patient had gone. Made several comments:

1. Overall praise for a job well done.

2. Omission of detailed explanation of test results was good. (This had been attempted during AA counseling without success.)

3. Explanation of trial rental evaluation was good. However, a suggestion: could have clarified difference between trial rental evaluation of h/a in *all* listening situations vs. later use on a selective basis. Gave sample of how this might be explained to patient.

4. Other suggestions:

    a. Further discussion of lipreading test results could have illustrated for patient the difference between unaided and aided listening while taking advantage of visual clues. (Later, listening to the tape, I discovered student had, in fact, done this—though it was probably not emphasized enough to the patient.)

    b. Need for continued lipreading with hearing aid could have been explained in more detail, again relating to test results, i.e., to non-visual listening (discrimination tests) vs. visual listening (Utley).

5. Response to patient's question about whether or not hearing aid use would be "nerve-wracking" was good.

6. Some comments made to student regarding the patient's reactions to our evaluation and the student's counseling.

7. Final discussion of hearing aid history picked up during the counseling session, its implications, and that it should be added to resumé.

APPENDIX III

EVALUATION WORKSHEET
FOR ROLE-PLAYING
SUPERVISION (sample)

In the audiology supervision course at Northwestern University, one of the class projects requires each student to supervise the course instructor as that instructor plays the role of a beginning clinical student (staff members are called upon to play the roles of patients). The "student" is to be supervised as though having had one practicum session preceding the current one. Following the session, evaluative comments, suggestions, and criticism are recorded by the course instructor in four areas and for each clinical activity. The grid used for this evaluation, with sample comments, is shown here.

Supervisory skill	Interview	Earphone, B/C oscillator placement; P/T test instructions	*Activity* Pure tone audiometry	Speech audiometry	Counseling[1]
	Prep. Thorough, appropriate review of history form. Step-by-step preparation with fairly good structure. (I helped structure it for you more than a real student would have done.) *During* Wisely took notes and did not intervene.	Earphones— You discussed/demonstrated earphone placement very well, but it probably would have been better had you explained it to me as I was doing it without first doing it yourself— just for the patient's sake. We could assume that you demonstrated it previously for me. B/C Oscillator—Good explanation of headband placement. Instructions— Excellent preparation. Good technique having me rehearse, then filling in the missing words.	*Prep.* Appropriate instruction regarding equipment setup: ear choice, starting level, frequency, etc. *During* Good step-by-step narration during threshold pursuit. *Post* Should have tied together reported symptoms with our findings better. Otitis media was mentioned, but what about associated allergies? And what about otosclerosis?	*Prep.* Fairly good setup of equipment. Not enough rationale explanation for controls. Sequencing of familiarization and instruction procedures was in reverse order.	*Prep.* Good nutshell preview of what you would cover in counseling. (This need not be done in detail since student will be listening anyway.) The important thing to explain—and you did this—is the rationale for counseling points and recommendations. Your biggest error here was not inviting me, the student, to observe your counseling so I could see how you used the audiogram, etc.
Knowledge of what to include in basic instruction for beginning student	*Post* Good suggestions for getting additional information (e.g., "people talk funny" implications; which ear otitis media was in), *but* why didn't you then have me or you ask these questions? Appropriately encouraged me before interview, and praised me afterwards. This was encouraging to me as a beginner.				

Clarity of explanation	Clarity of explanation generally quite good, though a little fuzzy on: chief complaint vs. reason for visiting clinic; and progression vs. fluctuation. Postinterview explanation of fluctuant hearing in association with overall normal sensitivity was a good point for me but a little advanced (and therefore confusing) for a beginning student.	Clarity of explanation excellent in all three of these areas. Comment: You told me to tell the patient she would be hearing tones in RE, then in LE. This is not a good idea.	Probably could have expanded your instructions to include a little more rationale. E.g., why do two correct responses on ascent constitute threshold? Why do we test RE first, then LE?	As a consequence, you had me give you practice test instructions, then practice familiarization instructions again. Your explanation/correction of instructions was good. Explanation of choosing sensation levels for discrimination was good but incomplete.	Your actual counseling was not as good as I know you probably can do. E.g., what did the patient mean when, after you showed her the B/C thresholds, she said, "I knew my hearing was normal!"?? Also, specific guidance regarding otologic consultation was not given until she initiated the discussion.
Detection of student's errors	The only blatant errors I made, and which you did not pick up, were: (1) I should have asked how long patient has noticed that people talk funny—this would have given us a clue as to time of onset; and (2) I should have asked whether or not there	Earphones—no great errors but you helped me re-seat the phones appropriately. B/C Oscillator—You missed it! I had the B/C vibrator on backwards (smooth side away from head). I thought you would discover it when you	You caught my depressing the interruptor switch for too long a time. You missed the fact that I did not take a correction factor into account at 2 kHz in the RE. As we discussed, you missed the earphone switch box missetting.	You caught my omission of certain equipment settings before I started talking to the "patient." You missed my underpeaking on the VU meter.	Not applicable

¹ Because this practicum assignment involved a beginning "student," the student supervisor was responsible for demonstrating the patient counseling portion of the audiologic evaluation.

Supervisory skill	Interview	Earphone, B/C oscillator placement; P/T test instructions	Activity Pure tone audiometry	Speech audiometry	Counseling[1]
	were any other family members with hearing loss following patient's report on mother.	repositioned it yourself, but you didn't. Instructions—no big errors, though my instructions were not smooth. (Would not expect them to be for beginners.)			
Ability to handle student's questions	You answered my questions well on dizziness vs. true vertigo, drugs vs. medication, and etiological significance of details in family history information.	I asked no questions in these areas.	Though I didn't ask, I presume you would have prepared me for pure tone masking. Your explanation of B/C oscillator placement on either mastoid, zero interaural attenuation, etc. was slightly confusing but a good start.	I didn't ask, but aren't there some conductives whose A/C configurations call for higher sensation levels than +26? I didn't ask (no beginner would have thought of it), but did you plan to mask for discrimination testing? You should have mentioned this when you discussed the preparatory steps.	Your postcounseling wrapup for me could have had a different, and more meaningful, emphasis if you hadn't been forced to explain to me the details of your audiogram explanation to the patient. In other words, again, I should have observed the counseling.

[1] Because this practicum assignment involved a beginning "student," the student supervisor was responsible for demonstrating the patient counseling portion of the audiologic evaluation.

APPENDIX IV

SAMPLE OUTLINE FOR REPORT OF SUPERVISORY EXPERIENCE

In the audiology supervision course for students at Northwestern University, a second class project (to take place after the one described in Appendix III) is the actual supervision of a first-year master's student working with an actual patient in an ongoing clinical activity. The student supervisors are evaluated on the quality of their written reports of this supervisory experience. The sample outline that is provided to guide them in report preparation is shown here.

I. Description of setting
   A. Status of student in clinical practicum
   B. Kind of clinical evaluation
   C. Place of clinical evaluation
   D. Type of case seen—brief description of patient problem (background and behavioral information, test findings, disposition of case)
II. Supervisory approach used
   A. Level(s) of supervision chosen, and rationale for selecting each, i.e., what kind of analytical thinking did you go through, and how did your resultant conclusions affect your choice of level(s)? Consider the following factors:
      1. Time allotment
      2. Difficulty of case
      3. Student knowhow
      4. Student speed
      5. Student/supervisor (you)/patient interaction
   B. Method of supervision—detailed explanation of supervisory steps employed (use Guide to Taped Supervision Sessions as example) from preevaluation instruction through postevaluation instruction
III. Overall evaluation of student's clinical skills, insofar as possible on the basis of this brief encounter
   Were the student's skills at a higher level than you expected of him at this stage in his clinical work, lower than your expectations, or commensurate with your expectations? Discuss the rationale for your answer
IV. Discuss your working relationship with the student
   A. How did the student seem to respond to your instruction—readily or reluctantly? Did he accept instruction without question? Ever disagree with you? How did his degree of responsiveness make you feel?
   B. Did you feel comfortable working with this student? He with you? Why or why not?
   C. Did student ask questions, make suggestions? Were they appropriate? How did you react? Was the dialogue between you and student meaningful, instructive?

V. Overall impression of supervisory experience
  A. Do you feel the student learned anything as a result of your supervision, i.e., do you think your supervision was effective? Why or why not?
  B. Did your supervisory experience alter your feelings about clinical supervision in any way? If so, how?
  C. Was this a valuable learning experience for you? Why or why not?

APPENDIX V

EVALUATION OF SUPERVISION/ CLINICAL PRACTICUM

This is a sample of the form currently used by students to evaluate supervisors, supervision, and practicum assignments in the Northwestern University audiology program. The first two general sections were designed to accommodate also the needs of students in comparable clinical areas.

Clinic_____

Supervisor_____Quarter/Year_____

Rate your supervision/clinical practicum experience only on items applicable to this particular assignment. For each item, complete the rating by circling the number of the descriptive term that reflects your closest appraisal of your clinical experience in terms of the following scale:

1. Unsatisfactory
2. Fair
3. Average
4. Good
5. Excellent

If you are unable to rate an item or it is not appropriate, circle "X" for the item.

CLINIC EVALUATION
Assess the value of this clinical assignment in terms of the experiences it offered in your overall educational program.

	Unsatis-factory	Fair	Average	Good	Excellent	Unable to rate or not appropriate
A. Appropriateness of this clinical practicum experience during the quarter in which it was assigned	1	2	3	4	5	X
B. Contribution of this practicum experience to your teaching/clinical competence	1	2	3	4	5	X
C. Effect of this clinical experience on your desire to become an audiologist/ teacher	1	2	3	4	5	X
D. Your overall rating of this clinical experience	1	2	3	4	5	X

Comments regarding clinical assignment _____

OVERALL EFFECTIVENESS OF SUPERVISION

Assess the following components of supervision in terms of their relative effectiveness in this assignment

		Unsatis-factory	Fair	Average	Good	Excellent	Unable to rate or not appropriate
A.	Explanation of clinical procedures	1	2	3	4	5	X
B.	Monitoring of your clinical work	1	2	3	4	5	X
C.	Amount and type of responsibility delegated to you	1	2	3	4	5	X
D.	Opportunity to express your own ideas on clinical work	1	2	3	4	5	X
E.	Freedom to ask questions of the supervisor	1	2	3	4	5	X
F.	Opportunity to implement your ideas	1	2	3	4	5	X
G.	Conduciveness of clinic atmosphere to your optimal performance	1	2	3	4	5	X
H.	Working relationship with your supervisor	1	2	3	4	5	X
I.	Supervisor's availability during clinic and nonclinic hours	1	2	3	4	5	X
J.	Supervisor's balancing of his/her obligation to the patient with his/her obligation to you	1	2	3	4	5	X
K.	Feedback on your clinical work and progress during the quarter	1	2	3	4	5	X
L.	Supervisor's evaluation of your performance	1	2	3	4	5	X
M.	Supervisor's clinical/educational skills	1	2	3	4	5	X

Comments regarding effectiveness of supervision _____

FOR CLINICAL PRACTICUM IN AUDIOLOGY

CLINICAL INSTRUCTION

Assess the supervisor's clinical instruction in terms of its content, manner of presentation, and effectiveness of presentation.

Specific test techniques

		Unsatis-factory	Fair	Average	Good	Excellent	Unable to rate or not appropriate
1.	Test instructions	1	2	3	4	5	X
2.	Pure tone audiometry	1	2	3	4	5	X
3.	Speech audiometry	1	2	3	4	5	X
4.	Masking	1	2	3	4	5	X
5.	Pediatric audiometry	1	2	3	4	5	X
6.	Impedance audiometry	1	2	3	4	5	X
7.	Use of test equipment	1	2	3	4	5	X

Hearing aids

		Unsatis-factory	Fair	Average	Good	Excellent	Unable to rate or not appropriate
1.	Preselection of hearing aids for clinic trial	1	2	3	4	5	X
2.	Hearing aid evaluation procedures	1	2	3	4	5	X

Resumés/reports

		Unsatis-factory	Fair	Average	Good	Excellent	Unable to rate or not appropriate
1.	Instruction regarding resumés and reports	1	2	3	4	5	X
2.	Editing and oral critique of written work	1	2	3	4	5	X

History taking

		Unsatis-factory	Fair	Average	Good	Excellent	Unable to rate or not appropriate
1.	Development of history taking skills	1	2	3	4	5	X
2.	Freedom allowed in asking your own questions and deviating from the history form	1	2	3	4	5	X

History taking

		Unsatis-factory	Fair	Average	Good	Excellent	Unable to rate or not appropriate
3.	Appropriateness of supervisor's intervention in your history taking	1	2	3	4	5	X
4.	Supervisory feedback on your history taking	1	2	3	4	5	X

Feedback/counseling

		Unsatis-factory	Fair	Average	Good	Excellent	Unable to rate or not appropriate
1.	Appropriateness of the amount of feedback/counseling responsibility given you	1	2	3	4	5	X
2.	Development of feedback/counseling skills	1	2	3	4	5	X
3.	Latitude allowed in incorporating your own thoughts into feedback/counseling	1	2	3	4	5	X
4.	Appropriateness of supervisor's intervention in your feedback/counseling	1	2	3	4	5	X
5.	Supervisor's followup instruction on your feedback/counseling	1	2	3	4	5	X

Special auditory test battery

		Unsatis-factory	Fair	Average	Good	Excellent	Unable to rate or not appropriate
1.	Test instructions	1	2	3	4	5	X
2.	Administration of tests	1	2	3	4	5	X
3.	Selection of appropriate tests	1	2	3	4	5	X
4.	Interpretation of tests and significance of test profiles	1	2	3	4	5	X
5.	Effectiveness of this clinical experience in expanding your understanding of the functions of a special auditory test battery	1	2	3	4	5	X

Effectiveness of instruction

	Unsatis-factory	Fair	Average	Good	Excellent	Unable to rate or not appropriate
1. Conformance of clinical instruction with your level of understanding	1	2	3	4	5	X
2. Structure in presentation of clinical concepts	1	2	3	4	5	X
3. Compatibility of information given in this assignment with that taught in your coursework	1	2	3	4	5	X
4. Compatibility of information given in this assignment with that given in your other clinical assignments	1	2	3	4	5	X

Comments regarding clinical instruction ⎯⎯⎯⎯⎯⎯⎯⎯⎯⎯⎯⎯⎯

APPENDIX VI

MINIMAL GOALS FOR STUDENTS

Some meetings of inservice training seminars for supervisors at Northwestern University were devoted to the formulation of minimal goals for expected student achievement in certain competency areas. Broad achievement goals, constructed for beginning, intermediate, and advanced proficiency levels, are shown here. (This entire form is currently under review by Northwestern University supervisors in their seminar deliberations on student evaluation.)

WORKING WITH ADULTS

Competency area	Expected achievement level		
	Beginner (1st quarter)	Intermediate (2d quarter)	Advanced (3d quarter or more)
Equipment	Knowledge of equipment operation. (Applies at all levels.) How and why of listening check.	Can troubleshoot equipment, detect problems.	Aware of equipment problems and appropriate solutions. Know where to turn for help in repair.
History taking	Able to determine what questions are appropriate after reviewing chart information, with supervisor help. Know what direction to go, with supervisor structure. Gross awareness of "red flag" markers of important information. Student expected to be "form bound."	History more student-directed, less supervisor structured. Better sense of appropriate questions, more student initiated. Know how to relate patient's symptoms to findings, interpretation and followup questions. Somewhat "form bound," mainly for internal structure.	Able to obtain history information independently, tell supervisor how history will be structured, and what questions will be asked. Greater flexibility, less "form bound." Able to field patient's questions.
Basic test skills Test instructions	Able to give instructions for a/c, b/c, SRT, discrimination. Beginning knowledge of masking instructions.	Able to give all instructions for conventional tests, though still need refinement. Continued work with masking instructions.	Know when and how to modify instructions in difficult cases.
Pure tone and speech audiometry	Proper placement of earphones and oscillator. Obtain pure tone audiogram on nonmasking cases, but aware of need for masking, and how much.	Refinement of basic AA skills, increasing speed with accuracy. Sense when modifications are needed. Able to obtain pure tone and	Continued refinement of skills with attention to speed and accuracy. Know when and how to modify test techniques in most difficult-to-test cases.

Obtain SRT in nonmasking cases, with supervisor structure. —Aware of PTA-SRT discrepancies. —Aware of need for masking, how much. Determine appropriate presentation level for discrimination, with moderate amount of supervisor structure for rationale. Knowledge of when to use full or half lists. Aware of need for masking for discrimination.	speech audiometry results on almost all cases. Able to explain rationale for each test step. Sense when evaluation is not proceeding as it should and when supervisor help is needed.	Independent in masking skills with infrequent supervision.
Impedance measurement Aware of what acoustic impedance measures. Obtain tympanograms and acoustic reflexes with constant supervision.	Obtain tympanograms and acoustic reflexes with moderate amount of supervision. Able to obtain hermetic seal in most cases.	Know difference between impedance bridge and otoadmittance meter. Obtain tympanograms and acoustic reflexes independently.
Interpretation of test results Developing awareness that composite results agree with one another and fit total picture. Developing awareness of test	Greater awareness of test result discrepancies and reasons for them, e.g., PTA-SRT disagreement, poor discrimination	(All of intermediate achievements with greater facility.) Able to interpret impedance findings independently.

continued

Key to abbreviations: AA—basic audiometric assessment for adult patients; D16-1—Principles of Audiologic Evaluation (first of a two-course sequence); D16-2—Principles of Audiologic Evaluation (second of a two-course sequence); STU—Special Test Unit.

Competency area	Expected achievement level		
	Beginner (1st quarter)	Intermediate (2d quarter)	Advanced (3d quarter or more)
	results and communicative implications.	Aware of test limitations. Better able to relate audiologic findings to suspected medical etiology and past history information. Awareness of various interpretations of masked pure tone responses, e.g., overmasking and mechanical artifacts. Awareness of impedance test interpretations. Awareness of "red flag" information that warrants further investigation.	Know when/how to modify test strategy.
Management and feedback	Observe supervisor manage.	Aware of what needs to be done and what needs to be said to the patient. Aware of everyday implications of test results. Provide feedback for normal hearing and more straightforward cases, with supervisor structure.	Provide feedback with structure provided mainly by student. Know what referrals need to be made. Know how to implement recommendations, with supervisor structure.
Resumés and reports	Summarize history and reason for referral. Describe audiometric findings. Summarize feedback and recommendations.	Improvement in writing style and use of terminology. More concise in summary.	Independent in writing skills with much less supervisory structure.

WORKING WITH CHILDREN

Competency area	Desired prerequisites		
	Beginner (1st quarter)	Intermediate (2nd quarter)	Advanced (3d quarter or more)
	Assume student has had adult AAs.	Assume student has had amplification course and one hearing aid clinic.	Previous or simultaneous assignment in diagnostic clinic helpful.
		Expected achievement level	
Test skills	Learn how to administer pediatric tests for sensitivity, discrimination and supplementary skills, i.e., CPA, VRA, BOA, WIPI, Peabody and Berry. Begin to develop understanding of rationale underlying test selection. Interpret earphone results, including impedance, on routine cases. (Does not include special sound field tests such as warble tones, VRA.) Familiarity with hearing aids *not* expected.	Know how to select the appropriate test technique. Know when/how to mask on routine cases. Begin to develop skills in modifying masking techniques for older children. Able to evaluate relationships among audiologic test findings (validity, reliability). Able to interpret sound field audiometric, and abbreviated earphone, findings. Develop familiarity with types of hearing aids. Able to: preselect and set hearing aid; do listening check on child's own hearing aid; put hearing aid on child; select appropriate tests for evaluation of aided	Able to work independently: should know what, how, when tests are to be done; should be able to interpret, while testing, results and their implications for abandonment of one technique in favor of others. Develop skills in modifying masking techniques for young children. Able to perceive relationships between test results and behavior/handicaps or skills as evaluation is progressing. Able to select appropriate hearing aid tests for younger children/nonroutine patients. Should be developing ability to generate subjective and objective findings, and give

continued

Competency area	Expected achievement level		
	Beginner (1st quarter)	Intermediate (2nd quarter)	Advanced (3d quarter or more)
		performance in older children. (All hearing aid skills dependent on clinical experience with adult hearing aid selections.) Develop basic behavior-shaping techniques needed to obtain auditory information, without supervisory direction. Able to observe and make informal judgments about motor, social and emotional development, and communicative skills.	rationale underlying decisions regarding amplification. Able to perceive child's response to test situation and modify own behavior in order to manage child's behavior. Able to make sophisticated overall observations.
Written work	Resumé and report to describe accurately history, routine audiologic findings and recommendations; major emphasis on audiologic sections. (Do *not* expect understanding or interpretation of additional observations, SF findings or hearing aid test results.)	Able to report accurately nonroutine, abbreviated, and/or SF findings. Report supplemental child and parental observations. Show developing awareness of relationships between child's handicaps and test findings and/or child's behavior, by end of quarter.	Able to write sophisticated, cohesive reports with awareness of dynamics and interrelationships. Reports should reflect any nonaudiologic recommendations. Reports should reflect differentiation according to intended recipient.

Interview/feedback	Interviews will be prestructured. Student expected to develop ability to gather information and know major history areas. (Do *not* expect development of any feedback skills.)	Able to develop histories differentially. Able to respond to, and explore, issues that arise during interview. Able to determine purpose of evaluation. **Begin** to develop ability to predict child's hearing status from interview. (Student to begin giving information-type feedback on routine cases, e.g., normal hearing or reevaluation with no significant change, if such cases arise.)	Continued development of more sophisticated interviewing skills. Feedback sessions to be done routinely by student unless case requires special management. Should be able to: convey audiologic information accurately; give clearcut audiologic recommendations (but not expected to give other types of management recommendations or information); begin developing responsiveness to issues and concerns that arise during feedback sessions.

HEARING AID PRACTICUM: ADULTS AND CHILDREN (See also Children, Test Skills)

Key: achievement levels (per student evaluation form)

3   Knows test techniques fairly well; requires moderate amount of supervision
4   Well informed on most aspects of testing; seldom requires assistance
5   Completely knowledgeable on all phases of testing; works independently

Competency area (per student evaluation form)	Expected achievement level		
	Beginner (1st quarter)	Intermediate (2d quarter)	Advanced (3d quarter, more)
Determination of amplification options, e.g.: Body-borne vs. ear level BTE vs. AIE vs. eyeglass Choice of ear to be aided Binaural, BICROS, CROS	3	4	5
Selection of individual aids, instrument settings, and earmold types, e.g.: Aids: gain, output, frequency response Molds: solid, modified (number, size of vents; length of canal tip; size of bore), open, no mold	3	3	4
Subjective evaluation skills, e.g.: Giving patient appropriate samples of speech to listen to (adequate quantity, modulation of voice, facial expression) Asking appropriate questions to determine patient's subjective reaction to sound quality and his comparative judgments Making appropriate decisions on basis of subjective information	3	4	4
Earmold fitting, volume setting skills, e.g.: Selecting (size/shape), inserting, removing earmolds correctly Selecting appropriate tubing Putting aid securely on patient Setting, adjusting volume controls appropriately	3	4	4
Trouble-shooting skills, e.g.: Identifying/isolating hearing aid problems via listening check and other means	3	3	4

Assessing patient's complaints regarding hearing aid sound quality, and dealing with them appropriately insofar as possible			
Solving feedback problems			
Selection of appropriate tests, e.g.: Knowing which tests to include, exclude, abbreviate	3	3	4
Knowing when to modify test procedures, e.g., MLV, dual scoring, elimination of carrier phrase, use of special test materials			
Interpretation of subjective and objective findings, and attendant decision making, e.g.:	3	3	4
Being able to assess findings throughout evaluation and make appropriate testing decisions			
Being able to integrate all available information (excluding dealer, price, referral source factors) at conclusion of evaluation and make appropriate recommendations			

SPECIAL TEST UNIT

Prerequisite: student has had D16-1; is in, or has had, D16-2.

Expected Achievement Levels at Beginning of STU Assignment

Demonstrated competency in all previous clinical assignments
Able to conduct AA independently
Have complete knowledge of masking and be able to apply it clinically

Desired Achievement Levels by Completion of STU Assignment

Able to conduct entire special test battery independently
Able to choose appropriate diagnostic tests for inclusion in battery
Able to interpret individual test results and test battery
Can explain results to physician, including indirect suggestions for further workups
Can make appropriate referrals for hearing aid investigation
Can write abbreviated letters with major conclusions highlighted for physician

The preceding set of goals for audiology students in clinical practicum is designed to be used as a *guideline* for supervisors. That is, modifications may be indicated, depending on the individual supervisor, the student, and the clinical assignment sequence.

Contributors are: Mary Burke, Sabina Kurdziel, Richard McCombs, Wynnette Moneka, Sheina Nicholls, Douglas Noffsinger, and Judith Rassi. These goals have been reviewed and discussed by the entire on-campus/off-campus supervisory staff of Northwestern University during the period from March to June, 1977.

APPENDIX VII

EVALUATION OF TRAINEES IN SUPERVISION PRACTICUM

The form used to evaluate the supervisors in training at Northwestern University, structured in content and format to conform with desirable supervisory characteristics, is shown here. Trainees are rated in each of the following areas, according to the scale displayed at the top of the form. Clinical competence and instruction skills in teaching ability are rated in each of the indicated areas; all other competencies are evaluated expressively.

KEY TO RATING SCALE

3—Good/Excellent
2—Fair/Adequate
1—Poor/Inadequate
Blank—Not evaluated or not applicable

CLINICAL COMPETENCE

Column headings (rating categories):
Clinic orientation; Equipment listening check; Equipment trouble-shooting; Review of medical charts and other information; Patient interview; Test instructions; Earphone, B/C oscillator placement; Pure tone audiometry; Masking; Speech audiometry; Impedance measurement; Counseling; Resumé/report writing

Rows:
Testing skills, knowhow
Independence in testing
Knowing when, how to deviate from routine procedures
Skill in interpreting implications (communicative, diagnostic) of test profile

TEACHING ABILITY

Instruction skills
1. Clarity of explanation
2. Accuracy of information

continued

3. Thoroughness in preparation of student for task

4. Thoroughness of topic coverage, underlying rationale

5. Ability to provide added insights, in-depth probes of clinical events

6. Ability to answer student's questions

Leadership

Ability to give direction and induce student to follow it in a firm but positive manner.

1. Constructiveness of criticism

2. Facility in helping student to improve areas of weakness

3. Appropriate amount/kind of praise for strengths, improvements

4. Approach in correcting student's errors

Communication

1. Encouragement of student to provide input

2. Receptiveness to student's suggestions

3. Appropriateness of verbal and body language

4. Appropriateness of model for student while communicating with patients

Interpersonal relationships

1. With student:
   a. Comfortableness in relating to student
   b. Flexibility in acceptance of different, but workable, methods

   c. Handling of differences in opinion
   d. Ability to detect, handle clinical personality problems
   e. Ability to perceive student attitudes, concerns
2. With patient
3. With supervising supervisor:
   a. Comfortableness in relating to supervising supervisor
   b. Compliance with supervising supervisor's suggestions, recommendations

Analysis

1. Ability to determine student's level(s) of proficiency and choose level(s) of supervision accordingly
2. Ability to analyze the clinical situation: student, patient, student/patient, time problems.

Facilitation

1. Ability to balance student's needs with patient's needs
2. Appropriateness of physical location, closeness of supervision

Management

1. Appropriateness/independence of patient management
2. Skill in management of time factors
3. Overall capacity to manage supervision responsibilities

Evaluation

1. Skill in detection of student errors
2. Overall proficiency in evaluation of student's:
   a. Clinical knowledge
   b. Clinical knowhow
   c. Clinical insight
   d. Clinical personality
3. Skill in editing student's written work
4. Ability to assess student's strengths and weaknesses
5. Handling of midterm evaluation conference
6. Final (written) evaluation:
   a. Appropriateness of rankings
   b. Insightfulness, thoroughness of comments
   c. Appropriateness of factors/judgments in determining final grade
   d. Handling of final evaluation conference with student

continued

Personal supervisory qualities

1. Patience
2. Sense of humor
3. Commitment to clinical supervision
4. Interest in continued learning in audiology, self-improvement in clinical skills
5. Flexibility
6. Emotional maturity
7. Common sense

IMPRESSION OF STUDENT'S RESPONSIVENESS TO SUPERVISOR/SUPERVISION

OVERALL PROGRESS OF SUPERVISOR SINCE BEGINNING OF SUPERVISION PRACTICUM

OVERALL EFFECTIVENESS OF SUPERVISION; POTENTIAL FOR SUPERVISORY WORK

REFERENCES

American Speech and Hearing Association. 1975a. News and announcements: Schools, hospitals, and clinics. Asha, 17, 238.

American Speech and Hearing Association. 1975b. Report of the legislative council: Supervision in speech pathology and audiology. Asha, 17, 175–176.

American Speech and Hearing Association. 1975c. Requirements for the Certificates of Clinical Competence.

American Speech and Hearing Association. 1975d. Your committees in action: Committee on supervision in speech pathology and audiology. Asha, 17, 397.

American Speech and Hearing Association. 1976a. ETB minimum requirements. Asha, 18, 110–113.

American Speech and Hearing Association. 1976b. Minimum requirements for ETB accreditation revised by ABESPA. Asha, 18, 318.

Anderson, J. L. (Ed.). 1970. Conference on Supervision of Speech and Hearing Programs in the Schools. Bloomington, Ind.: Indiana University.

Anderson, J. L. 1972. Status of supervision of speech, hearing, and language programs in the schools. Lang. Speech Hear. Serv. Schools, 3:1, 12–22.

Anderson, J. L. 1973a. Status of college and university programs of practicum in the schools. Asha, 15, 60–65.

Anderson, J. L. 1973b. Supervision: The neglected component of our profession. In L. J. Turton (Ed.), Proceedings of a Workshop on Supervision in Speech Pathology, pp. 4–28. Ann Arbor, Michigan: University of Michigan, Institute for the Study of Mental Retardation and Related Disabilities, Continuing and Adult Education Unit.

Anderson, J. L. 1974. Supervision of school speech, hearing, and language programs—an emerging role. Asha, 16, 7–10.

Anderson, J. L. 1975. Clinical supervision: Issues and practices. Paper presented at the North Central Regional Conference of the American Speech and Hearing Association, May, Minneapolis.

Barnhart, C. L. (Ed.). 1968. The Random House American Dictionary and Family Reference Library. New York, New York: Random House, Inc.

Blumberg, A. 1974. Supervisors and Teachers: A Private Cold War. Berkeley, California: McCutchan Publishing Corp.

Boone, D. R., and Prescott, T. E. 1972. Content and sequence analyses of speech and hearing therapy. Asha, 14, 58–62.

Brown, E. L. 1967. A university's approach to improving supervision. In A. Miner (Ed.), A symposium: Improving supervision of clinical practicum. Asha, 9, 476–479.

Brown, E. L. 1975. Clinical supervision: Issues and practices. Paper presented at the North Central Regional Conference of the American Speech and Hearing Association, May, Minneapolis.

Brown, E., Anderson, J., Dublinske, S., and Herbert, E. 1972. Task force report on supervision in the schools. Lang. Speech Hear. Serv. Schools, 3:3, 4–10.

Carhart, R., and Jerger, J. 1959. Preferred method for determining pure-tone threshold. J. Speech Hear. Disord., 24, 330–345.

Cogan, M. L. 1973. Clinical Supervision. Boston: Houghton Mifflin.

Culatta, R., Colucci, S., and Wiggins, E. 1975. Clinical supervisors and trainees: Two views of a process. Asha, 17, 152–157.

Culatta, R., and Seltzer, H. 1976. Content and sequence analysis of the supervisory session. Asha, 18, 8–12.

Culatta, R., and Seltzer, H. 1977. Content and sequence analysis of the supervisory session: A report of clinical use. Asha, 19, 523–526.

Curlee, R. F. 1975. Personal incomes in the speech and hearing profession. Asha, 17, 21–30.

Darley, F. L. (Ed.). 1963. Graduate Education in Speech Pathology and Audiology: Report of a National Conference. Washington, D.C.: American Speech and Hearing Association.

Darley, F. L. 1969. Clinical training for full-time clinical service: A neglected obligation. Asha, 11, 143–148.

Engnoth, G. L., and Lingwall, J. B. 1974. A comparison of three approaches to supervision of speech clinicians in training. Paper presented at the Annual Convention of the American Speech and Hearing Association, November, Las Vegas.

Erickson, J. G., and Garstecki, D. C. 1973. Practicum in aural rehabilitation in a university training program. J. Acad. Rehab. Audiol., 6, 9–12.

Erickson, R., and Van Riper, C. 1967. Demonstration therapy in a university training center. Asha, 9, 33–35.

Gerstman, H. L. 1977. Supervisory relationships: Experiences in dynamic communication. Asha, 19, 527–529.

Goldhammer, R. 1969. Clinical Supervision. New York: Holt, Rinehart and Winston.

Gordon, T. 1974. T.E.T. Teacher Effectiveness Training. New York: David McKay Company, Inc.

Halfond, M. 1964. Clinical supervision—Stepchild in training. Asha, 6, 441–444.

Hood, J. D. 1960. Principles and practices of bone-conduction audiometry. Laryngoscope, 70, 1211–1228.

Ingram, D. B., and Stunden, A. A. 1967. Student's attitude toward the therapeutic process. Asha, 9, 435–441.

Jerger, J. 1974. Forum: The future of audiology. Asha, 16, 249–250.

Kleffner, F. (Ed.). 1964. Seminar on Guidelines for the Internship Year. Washington, D.C.: American Speech and Hearing Association.

Klevans, D. R., and Volz, H. B. 1974. Development of a clinical evaluation procedure. Asha, 16, 489–491.

Knepflar, K. J. 1976. Report Writing in the Field of Communication Disorders. Danville, Ill.: The Interstate Printers and Publishers, Inc.

Miner, A. (Ed.). 1967. A symposium: Improving supervision of clinical practicum. Asha, 9, 471–481.

Minifie, F. D. 1975. Is my future secure? Keynote address presented at the North Central Regional Conference of the American Speech and Hearing Association, May, Minneapolis.

Mullendore, J. M., and Koller, D. E. 1976. The elements of contemporary supervision. Paper presented at the Annual Convention of the Illinois Speech and Hearing Association, April, Chicago.

Muma, J. R., Mann, M. B., and Trenholm, S. A. 1976. Training programs in speech pathology and audiology: Demographic data, perceived departmental and personal functions, and productivity. Asha, 18, 419–432, 445–446.

Oratio, A. R. 1977. Supervision in Speech Pathology. A Handbook for Supervisors and Clinicians. Baltimore: University Park Press.

Pannbacker, M. 1975. Diagnostic report writing. J. Speech Hear. Disord., 40, 367–379.

Pickering, M. 1977. An examination of concepts operative in the supervisory process and relationship. Asha, 19, 607–610.

Rees, M., and Smith, G. L. 1967. Supervised school experience for student clinicians. Asha, 9, 251–256.

Rees, M., and Smith, G. L. 1968. Some recommendations for supervised school experience for school clinicians. Asha, 10, 93–103.

Rosen, J. 1967. Distortions in the training of audiologists. Asha, 9, 171–174.

Schubert, G. W. 1974. Suggested minimal requirements for clinical supervisors. Asha, 16, 305.

Schubert, G. W., and Aitchison, C. J. 1975. A profile of clinical supervisors in college and university speech and hearing training programs. Asha, 17, 440–447.

Schultz, M. C. 1972. An Analysis of Clinical Behavior in Speech and Hearing. Englewood Cliffs, N.J.: Prentice-Hall.

Schultz, M. C. 1975. Clinical decision making. Miniseminar presented at the Annual Convention of the American Speech and Hearing Association, November, Washington, D.C.

Shriberg, L. D., Bless, D. M., Carlson, K. A., Filley, F. S., Hayes, D. M., Kwiatkowski, J., and Smith, M. E. 1975a. Forum: Research in supervision. Asha, 17, 792.

Shriberg, L. D., Filley, F. S., Hayes, D. M., Kwiatkowski, J., Schatz, J. A., Simmons, K. M., and Smith, M. E. 1975b. The Wisconsin procedure for appraisal of clinical competence (W-Pacc): Model and data. Asha, 17, 158–165.

Stace, A. C., and Drexler, A. B. 1969. Special training for supervisors of student clinicians: What private speech and hearing centers do and think about training their supervisors. Asha, 11, 318–320.

Starkweather, C. W. 1974. Behavior modification in training speech clinicians: procedures and implications. Asha, 16, 607–611.

Tillman, T. W., and Olsen, W. O. 1972. Speech audiometry. In J. Jerger (Ed.), Modern Developments in Audiology. (2nd ed.) New York: Academic Press.

Turton, L. J. (Ed.). 1973. Proceedings of a Workshop on Supervision in Speech Pathology. Ann Arbor, Mich.: Univ. of Michigan, Institute for the Study of Mental Retardation and Related Disabilities, Continuing and Adult Education Unit.

Ulrich, S. R., and Giolas, T. G. 1977. Status of clinical supervisors: A model for reappointment and promotion. Paper presented at the Annual Convention of the American Speech and Hearing Association, November, Chicago.

Unruh, A., and Turner, H. E. 1970. Supervision for Change and Innovation. Boston: Houghton Mifflin.

Van Riper, C. 1965. Supervision of clinical practice. Asha, 7, 75–77.

Van Riper, C., and Dopheide, W. 1966. Diagnostic services in a training center. Asha, 8, 37–39.

Villareal, J. J. (Ed.). 1964. Seminar on Guidelines for Supervision of Clinical Practicum in Programs of Training for Speech Pathologists and Audiologists. Washington D.C.: American Speech and Hearing Association.

Ward, L. M., and Webster, E. J. 1965a. The training of clinical personnel: I. Issues in conceptualization. Asha, 7, 38–40.

Ward, L. M., and Webster, E. J. 1965b. The training of clinical personnel: II. A concept of clinical preparation. Asha, 7, 103–106.

AUTHOR INDEX

SUBJECT INDEX